Yoga Diet

Lose weight Fast

How to lose 10 pounds in 10 DAYS with Yoga?

by

Sammy Hermans

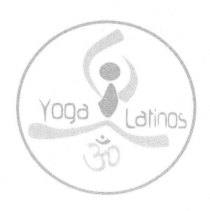

Copyright

How will this book benefit YOU?

Are you ready for all the benefits this book can bring to Your life? Discover why you must read this book and start with the 10 days Yoga Diet program from Today:

- You will Start losing weight from Day 1 with this amazing Yoga Diet,
- Your body will have more energy for during the day,
- Become more flexible with the basic Yoga poses,
- Reward yourself with this healthy diet that makes you feel Great all Day,
- After 10 days your body will be detoxed,
- Get Stress relief thanks to this program,
- You're confidence level will go up,
- Feel better mentally and physically,
- Start to learn who you really are thanks to this book,
- Be ready to enjoy life at his maximum.

Contents

Thank You

I would like to begin this book by thanking you to read one of the books I have written to change your life. I know your time is valuable and I am very grateful that you decided to take a little time out of your day to read my book. I am sure you will be happy with the results after following the 10 days Yoga program.

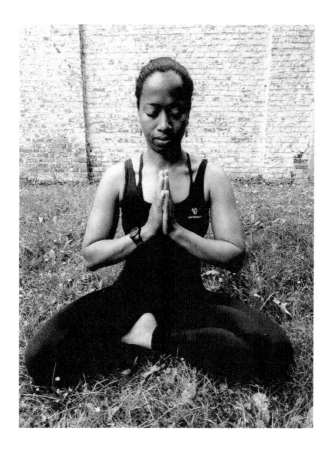

The author

Sammy Hermans is an upcoming author that was born in the early 80's and has since childhood a great interest in the Yoga art. He was studying multiple Yoga styles and grew up in Belgium, the capital of Europe. The author is a real world citizen and likes to get new influences from all over the world.

The author loves to do research about the different Yoga styles to implement them in the Yoga classes and help people to find the best Yoga styles that fits them. Meditation has helped him gain control over his mind and live a stress-free, more productive, healthy and happier life. Sammy enjoys seeing the wonderful improvements in peoples lives through yoga. He loves to help people with this new lifestyle and guide them through this healthy journey. The author is always willing to help people to become happier and healthier.

The author started a Yoga training and Yoga coaching business together with his partner Sherley Henry De Hermans. The company 'Yoga Latinos' was created to help people along their journey towards a healthy Yoga life. Together they are willing to help and guide everybody in their new mindset. Please check out www.yogalatinos.com if you are interested in more Yoga information on the blog or if you are interested in online Yoga classes.

Sammy's other interests include world music, dancing, relaxing and meditation, multimedia arts, reading, traveling, spending time in nature & drinking cups of tea and enjoying time with his wife, kids and family.

Discover all the amazing ideas in his books.

Prologue: Why I wrote the 10 DAYS program?

On many occasions, we try to do exercises that are rigorous in order to lose weight. We sometimes try aggressive plans, although it can be dangerous for some people. But, who said losing weight should be a painful process?

It should be a process that we long to undergo every stipulated time. We should not dread the time that we engage our bodies in these exercises. It is based on this that I developed the 10 days Yoga exercises and diet. After going through many exercises and reading on different diet combinations, I came up with a plan that covered the major diets and exercises that have been recommended by leading nutritionists.

I am confident that if you stick to the plan, you will burn that fat that has been refusing to go away. The diet is one element that is equally important with the Yoga exercises when trying to lose weight. There is a need to blend different diets for maximum results. Different diets are effective on different levels. This Yoga diet is everything you need.

Are you tired with the daily routine workouts that you engage your body every day? The truth is that in order to be efficient in our workout plans, we need to switch the daily workouts so that the body will be challenged. Many people who have lost hope in exercising, either going to the gym, or doing outdoor activities, get used to the routine that they go through every day. Doing Yoga will give you new energy to move your body.

Our bodies have been programmed to get accustomed to something and when this is reached, you need to look for some new routine. When our bodies reach the stage where they are accustomed to some workout, they will no longer work hard to do what it has been doing every day. At this stage, there is nothing new that is achieved. We never get benefits in terms of muscle development, strength enhancement, and general weight loss.

The solution to this is to have a blend of exercises and diets. It is a no-string attached kind of weight loss program. We should adopt a different approach to exercises and diets. We should try to learn the various exercises, and diets and what benefits they have on our bodies. With this approach, our bodies will lose weight fast because the workouts hit the muscles in different angles, and in different intensities. It is also beneficial because one's flexibility, speed, and balancing of the body will be improved. It is a fast way of losing excess fat and enhancing the strength of the muscles.

Blending different types of workouts can be compared to treatment of the body with shock; it kills the boredom, and eliminates laziness and monotony. These benefits can also be said about the foods, that is, we will not be bored with taking one type of food days on end.

The program has been developed with the mindset that the cardiovascular routine workouts should be changed as well. We have to change the way we perceive cardiovascular exercises. We should use different machines or have different outdoor activities so that we are flexible even in the cardiovascular exercises. As has been stated above, blending exercises will help work on the different parts of the body. A split routine is a workout plan which will follow different workouts for different parts of the body. The program targets the different parts of the body in that it balances the straining because not one part of the body will be overworked.

This program was developed for people who have been doing workouts continuously. It is also good for starters, but after they have stretched their bodies so that the bodies are already prepared for exercises. It is a comprehensive program that you should start immediately in order to get results as soon as possible. With time, even starters will eventually develop the endurance level, and the stamina that is required to manage a blend of workouts.

As this program follows the no-string-attached approach to exercising, new beginners should take caution so that they are not injured.

You might notice that in the book the word "yoga" is always written with a capital Y, as in Yoga. This is because Yoga have to become a mindset for you. By reading the word "Yoga", your mind will unconsciously remember, what will give you more motivation to follow the Yoga lifestyle.

 It is a program you cannot afford to miss. It is comprehensive, wholesome, and tested! Its an innovative program that will ensure that you lose 10 pounds after the 10th day!

The bottom-line is, in order to enhance the strength of the body, and continuously challenge the body, try this 10 days program.

You will not turn to any other weight losing program if you follow this program.

Chapter 1: Can the 10 DAYS program really work for me?

Many people believe that weight loss arises from excessively strict dieting, strenuous cardio and even weight training; Yoga may frequently be overlooked as an option for weight loss as it is not commonly thought of as a slimming exercise.

However, Yoga should be considered for weight loss as there are many benefits to participating in this exercise. Yoga allows for participants to strengthen their inner core muscles and build strength. Whilst this form of exercise may not burn an extensive amount of calories, it allows for the individual to train their mind to make healthier choices.

This new way of healthier thinking promotes healthy choices relating to the individual's body, such as the decision to eat healthier foods and participate in more regular physical activity.

Whilst Yoga traditionally does not burn the calories that walking or running does, Yoga helps a person increase their own mindfulness, particularly how they think of and relate to their own self and body.

For example, regular participation in Yoga allows one to develop a deep sense of understanding about their body, and even a connection with themselves and their health. An avid Yoga participant will be aware of how they are feeling internally, and additionally will understand what foods make their body feel better or worse. This will help to promote healthier choices in relation to the consumption of certain foods; therefore, Yoga, through promoting an awareness of self, promotes healthy eating choices and therefore weight loss.

A common question posed by many who are unfamiliar with Yoga and the related benefits is often "can Yoga really work for me?" The answer is simple: **YES!** Yoga can work for anyone who is open to participating in an activity that will allow the person to relate to and connect with their body. "Can this 10 days Yoga food and Yoga exercise program work for me?" The answer is **YES!**

Here's why: primarily, Yoga involves continuous use of your muscles, which burns calories. This means that your muscles are continuously stretching and working, which means you are exercising, which in turn promotes weight loss. So, as a result, this aspect of participating in the activity alone means Yoga will work for you as a form of weight loss!

Furthermore, this program only requires 15 minutes of Yoga exercise per day, so it's easy to participate and get motivated!

The second aspect of this 10 days program is the food. Following this diet that has been provided to you will not only decrease your calorie intake to a healthier level, but will also promote an increase in your metabolism, thus enhancing weight loss. Weight loss typically occurs when a person's calorie intake is less than their calorie expenditure. Simply put, if you burn more calories than you eat, your body will be forced to burn its own fat storage, causing you to lose weight.

The foods chosen in this 10 days Yoga food and Yoga exercise program are designed to work in combination with a Yoga exercise program to maximize your weight loss! The particular foods have been proven to satisfy hunger and cravings even though they are low in calories; the perfect combination for weight loss!

Furthermore, the food chosen for this Yoga food and Yoga exercise program are portioned in realistic sizes, unlike many other diets that leave you feeling hungry. After reading the book you should be able to learn more about your own body and feel when to stop eating; in order to avoid eating too many calories.

This program considers the individual; foods have been chosen that are tasty and won't make you feel like you're on a 10 days diet. Most people may even continue the food plan after the 10 days because it is a realistic way that is not a diet, but a lifestyle and a way of eating healthier. The results speak for themselves and you will see these results yourself after your 10 days participation!

In conclusion, will this program work for you? The answer is, **Yes.** This 10 days Yoga food and Yoga exercise program will have you connect with your inner self and make healthier choices that promote weight loss. This program will promote daily exercise to tone and tighten your body in combination with a diet that will speed up your metabolism and burn fat.

The program will work for you because even from day 1 you will feel as though you are not on a diet or completing a rigorous exercise scheme, but rather you are making a life change to improve your overall health and well being; what could possible feel better than that?

Chapter 2:Do you weigh too much?

Many people are not sure if they weigh too much. They may think they are overweight in comparison to what they see in the media. The following are some metrics on how to determine whether you weigh too much, and by how much.

Your significant other tells you:

Has your significant other been making jokes that you are looking a little more heavy lately? Chances are, they are telling the truth. Not to be taken offensively, but your significant other is probably telling you this information because they care about you, and want you to be healthy.

Most people have a difficult time telling their friends or colleagues that they are concerned about their weight, so one of the more honest sources is your significant other.

Limited closet choices:

Do you find that all of a sudden you have limited clothes to wear for work or to go out? Your clothes are not disappearing, but you have run out of options that fit.

Rather than go to the store to buy more clothes, it might be time to consider that you weigh too much, and it is time to do something about it. Follow the 10 days program and start to wear your favorite clothes again.

Fewer people want to talk to you:

If you are single, and you frequently visit bars or nightclubs, fewer people might try to talk to you. The unfortunate matter of being overweight, is that society places increased pressure on people to be thin or fit in order to be desirable. You may realize that you have put on too much weight when you notice that fewer people have tried to ask for your phone number, or have tried to flirt with you when you are out.

Although this might be because of a shallow person, you might consider that overweight is a problem for your social improvement. After following the 10 days program and changing your lifestyle, you might notice that your social contacts will improve and increase.

Physical exertion:

Another way to determine if you weigh too much is if you are having a difficult time with physical exertion. If walking up the stairs is becoming very difficult for you, to the point that you are out of breath, you might weigh too much.

Additionally, if you find that you cannot run around and play games with your children (or other kids) or you can't walk far distances like you used to, these may be indicators that it is time to lose some weight.

Consult with your doctor:

One of the best ways to determine if you weigh too much is to speak to your primary care doctor about it. Not only can your doctor conduct take your weight to see if it is within a healthy range, but your doctor can also conduct additional tests to determine if you are having health issues related to being overweight.

You may have your blood taken for cholesterol and fasting blood sugar screening to determine if you are at risk for developing heart disease or diabetes, two illnesses that are associated with being overweight.

Chapter 3: What is BMI?

The concept of Body Mass Index (BMI) was adopted by Adolphe Quetelet, a Belgian astronomer, statistician, mathematician, and sociologist. Initially called the "Adolphe Index", this calculation was originally used to track the growth process of man. He noted that one's weight tends to increase with their height at a certain pace, and he wanted to track the rate of that pace.

Today, people use a tweaked version of this index to check for trends in weight and healthy lifestyles. Body Mass Index (BMI) is a way to derive the percentage of body fat given an individual's height and weight. Body mass index, also known as BMI, is an assessment of a person's weight in kilograms in comparison to their height in meters.

The BMI can also be an indicator of a person's body fat in comparison to their height, however, since everyone's proportion of fat and muscle are different, BMI should only be used as a guideline in collaboration with other measures.

The formula for BMI is: weight (kg) / [height (m)]^2. However, there are several online resources to easily assist you in calculating your BMI. Simply enter in your weight, and height, and you can interpret your BMI from there.

BMI is classified under four categories: underweight, normal weight, overweight, and obese. As told above the BMI is defined by the weight of an individual (in kg) divided by their height squared (in meters). The equation is seen as kg/m^2.

But people using the Imperial units of measurement find their body mass index by taking their weight in pounds multiplied by 703, then dividing the product by the square of their height in inches. This system is used by doctors using the Imperial units of measurement to determine if someone is underweight, normal-weight, overweight or obese.

Someone who is underweight will typically have a BMI of below 18.5. Normal BMI ranges from 18.5 - 25. Someone who is overweight will usually have a BMI of 25-30. Anyone with a BMI over 30 is considered obese.

 BMI is an easy way to reference whether you are over, or underweight. While it has its limitations, it is an easy way to reference body weight and body fat with the general population.

On average, people with a BMI of 18.4 and below are at higher risk of developing nutritional deficiencies and osteoporosis in their lifetime. People with a BMI between

18.5 - 22.9 are considered to be in the "normal zone", and are thus at low risk for dietary related illnesses. Those with a BMI between 23.0 and 27.4 are said to be at "moderate risk" of developing heart disease, high blood pressure, stroke, and diabetes. Those with a BMI of 27.5 and above are at high risk of the previous ailments.

There are a few people that can not get an accurate reading from BMI calculations : infants, athletes and the elderly. Athletes weigh more because of their high muscle mass. Infants cannot be accurately measured based on height and weight, and the elderly tend to lose muscle over time, thus making their weight decrease.

 BMI is a relatively simple way to understand one's body and to quickly check one's body-weight, but it does have its limitations.

Firstly, BMI calculations cannot differentiate fat from muscle weight. Someone who is lighter but has a higher fat content may have a lower calculated BMI than someone who is heavier because they have more muscle mass. That is why athletes cannot accurately test their BMI using these calculations. People can weigh more but have as little as 5% body fat, simply because their body is mostly heavy muscle.

The BMI calculations are not a perfect way to determine where you are at in terms of health, it can serve as a decent guideline. There are other important factors to keep in mind when calculating BMI. These include things like skin fold thickness, dietary habits, exercise habits, age, and family health history.

Some people can easily appear to be overweight when they should be considered "normal". Likewise, those who are overweight may not be able to detect it with these calculations. BMI should be viewed more in a way to view trends in populations, rather than individuals. It is important to consult with a doctor or dietitian about your health and eating habits, before jumping to conclusions about weight.

BMI machines can help give a more accurate reading of body fat percentage. They work by sending a small electrical signal through both of your hands. While this doesn't hurt at all, it is very important to tracking body fat. The electrical signal travels through water. Unlike muscle, fat has little to no water in it. Therefore, the longer it takes for the electrical signal to travel, the more body fat the machine detects. Doctors say that the machine works best in the morning, when you already drink water. That way, the machine won't mistake dehydration for high fat content.

Again, while all of these resources are helpful, nothing beats checking with a doctor or nutritionist to ensure that you are on a healthy track. Weight can be a good indicator of health, but it isn't everything.

Body Fat Composition Analysis with Calipers:

Since BMI is not the only way to assess whether you weigh too much, you can also do this, as told above, with a body fat composition analysis with calipers. A caliper is a device used to measure the amount of fat in your skin folds. You can have this process done at a gym, personal trainer, nutritionist, or even your doctor. There are body fat calipers available for purchase online, and you can learn how to measure your body fat on different websites that have quick tutorials on how to measure your body fat based on your gender, and a lot of times there is a calculator where you can determine your body fat composition.

There are several ways to determine if you weigh too much.

If you realize that you weigh too much, have no fear. Read on to learn more about how to lose 10 pounds in 10 DAYS with Yoga.

Chapter 4: The basic principles of Yoga exercises

It is said that if you cannot explain something in simple terms, then you simply don't understand it. I could say that when it comes to Yoga, this truth holds a lot of water. What would be the point of carrying out all the Yoga exercises day in day out if you don't understand the very principles behind them? To this end, it is important to go back to the very basics. What principles lie behind Yoga exercises?

What is proper breathing?:

You might think you know how to breathe until you try out the deep, rhythmic and slow breaths as is required during Yoga breathing exercises. Breathing might often seem like an effortless body process but it should be done properly.

What then is proper breathing? Well, this has to do with embracing correct breathing techniques. Breathing in and out through the nose with lengthened exhalations would be a good place to start, followed by a short pause to induce a state of tranquility.

Proper breathing requires you to breathe with your whole body, something that people are not doing as often due to being too conscious of their surroundings. Have you seen how a newborn baby breathes? How their tummies rise and fall with each inhale and exhale when they are asleep? This is what proper breathing is all about.

Correct breathing should have you push out the abdomen while inhaling for maximum lung expansion and then letting it come back in naturally while exhaling. When we breathe with the whole body, it gives the entire body some sort of massage that works to soothe all the body organs down to the tiny cells. Taking in deep slow breaths will help clear your lungs of stale air and provide rich oxygen that is required by the body. The diaphragmatic breathing should have your diaphragm rise and fall with every breath with an exhale almost two times longer than the inhale.

The whole point of these proper breathing techniques is to increase the uptake of oxygen by the lungs. This to energize the body through maximization of oxygen presence in the blood and to seize control of the mind through regulation of the flow of the life force, which is the air we breathe.

Proper breathing enables you to properly take up the vital energy that is air and distribute it through our entire body. What's more is that the controlled breathing enables you to have a calmer, clearer and focused mind. Proper breathing is all about breathing long and deeply to maximize the capacity of the lungs.

What is proper dieting?:

For all of you out there looking to shed off some of that extra weight, 70% of the process has to do with your food habits. Yes. Don't be a slave to your taste buds. You are literally what you eat!

The food you eat is what builds up your body. So what then is a proper diet? Simply put, it should be one that nourishes body and mind. If you want, you can forget about the laborious task of counting calories, it all depends on the quality of the food. Forget about what it tastes like, focus more on the nutritional value of the food you take. Did you know that the kind of food you take has an impact on your mental capacity?

Poor diets that lack nutrients are detrimental to our brains leading to depression and anxiety. Yoga exercises should place you on a path of proper dieting whereby moderation guides all your food choices. The recommended food quantity should have you only fill half your stomach with food, a quarter of the stomach with water and the remaining quarter should be empty to provide ample space for digestion to take place.

This is a great way to do the diet without counting calories, although for maximum results you should measure what you eat. But by following the 10 days program, only relying on the half fill stomach rule, you will already see incredible results.

Water should be taken at least thirty minutes before a meal. Eat only when hungry to avoid comfort eating and general overeating which end up heavily taxing your digestive system for nothing, leaving you sluggish and under active. Opt for fresh, organic and nutritious food derived from nature such as milk, honey, fruits and vegetables that are easy to digest. Fresh food should therefore be preferably prepared by oneself to know what exactly goes into making it.

Avoid frozen, canned, spicy, oily, stale, chemically enhanced, refined grains and refined sugar types of food that are a common characteristic of fast foods that are high on cholesterol and save your heart the trouble of a probable heart disease.

Chewing food properly enables it to be easily assimilated for purposes of digestion. Proper dieting should have you adopt a vegetarian diet that is built on grain and vegetable intake, which take a few hours to be digested and to exit the system.

Meat, alcohol, eggs, artificially flavored, chemically processed and enhanced foods are discouraged usually because they take longer to digest, therefore, overworking the digestive system using up a lot of energy while being least beneficial to the body and mind.

They also lower body immunity when taken in excess. Make sure to partake of a balanced diet consisting of vegetables, herbs, legumes, nuts, fiber and carbohydrates together with small portions of oil and raw sugar. These are easily digestible and promote good health and provide energy. Always remember that we eat to live, but do not live to eat.

What is proper exercising?:

Yoga exercises and poses, known as asanas, provide a myriad of positions to help in moving your entire body. These poses help in exercising your body by engaging your core to stabilize the body. What's even better about Yoga exercises, is that they do so much for you at once.

They not only strengthen, tone and lengthen muscles and ligaments, but also raise the heartbeat. Proper exercises means that you get to do a variety of fun poses with zero chances of injury. This means you get to enjoy the Yoga exercises to the fullest. Talk about hitting two birds with one stone!

Proper exercises are also meant to ensure your mind and spirit are exercised as well to broaden their capacities. Proper yogic exercises usually focus on the spine to enhance its flexibility and strength to help improve on circulation of nutrients and oxygen throughout the body. The internal organs such as heart as well as glands and hormones are also affected by asanas to ensure they are properly functioning.

Asanas generally range from arm balances to inversions to back bends that work on specific body parts such as lower back to hamstrings. These exercises work to tackle different ailments such as insomnia and headaches. In general however, Yoga exercises work to gain strength and flexibility all at once through the steady poses that should be conducted slowly and consciously.

These proper exercises work best when coordinated with breaths, making them one and more beneficial, not only to physical strength but also to mental and spiritual growth. The asanas should be done quietly and in a particular order that allow for the systematic movement of every part of the body to enhance the life force of energy.

Yoga exercises improves on balance through strengthening the lower body, the ankles and knees in particular. The exercises also reduce general mobility problems through promotion of strength and flexibility.

For those seeking to lose weight, fat burning Yoga poses and workouts that not only strengthen the core, but also shed off love handles and tone the buttocks along with the inner and outer thighs.

What is proper relaxation?:

Relaxation is a skill that should be mastered by all since there is no better way to cool down and re-energize your body. Relaxation works to loosen body and mental tension. Deep and proper relaxation rejuvenates the nervous system, boosts efficiency of body systems and helps one achieve a sense of tranquility.

Yoga exercises strive to ensure that mind and body are not constantly overworked and provide for a recharge system through relaxation. Even while relaxation might come about as an effortless activity to many, it needs to be properly mastered to ensure none of our energy goes to waste.

Foul moods are often very consuming and a slight moment of anger and irritation usurp our much needed energy, especially if a habit is made out of such moods thus proving to be disastrous. Proper relaxation should have you without any form of tension whatsoever to ensure no amount of energy is being consumed. To this end, relaxation should be physical, mental and spiritual for it to count as proper relaxation.

Physical relaxation should have you clear your mind of any thoughts which might result in your body taking action. All body muscles should be relaxed to attain a state of actual relaxation where there is no muscular tension almost as if lifeless. Conscious relaxation will train your muscles to release their grip when you don't use them.

Mental relaxation should have you steer clear of any kind of external thought while breathing slowly to get rid of the tension and switch to a state of self-awareness whereby you are in control. Rhythmic breathing helps clear the mind and body quite easy.

Spiritual relaxation will be attained by connecting to a higher power to whom we connect with for spiritual ease and relief over things we don't have control over. Spiritual relaxation enables one to withdraw oneself from the body and mind to get rid of emotions such as anxiety, fear, worry and sorrow that bring about tension.

All these combined lead to a true state of relaxation and help in stress management. Relaxation is also a working remedy that works for individuals who want to lose weight without necessarily having to go on a diet. Relaxation is a Yoga exercise principle that works to aid in weight reduction by reducing the cravings for unhealthy foods that result in weight gain due to the empty calories contained in them.

Relaxation is linked to better food and lifestyle choices that are not related to stress such as binge eating thus aiding in significant weight loss.

What is positive thinking and meditation?:

Yoga is a mental discipline. What you think, you become! Therefore, direct the mind the right way. Yoga teaches on importance of striving to think of good things that are not only positive but creative. With the possible blows that life might deal you, it is imperative to maintain that positive outlook.

One should steer clear of mental agitation by shifting focus from all that is around towards one's own self to achieve maximum concentration to achieve a state of meditation.

Positive thinking should have one fine-tune their minds to always look at the positive side of things. For those seeking to lose weight, it all begins in the mind. Overeating is usually linked to self-loathing which builds up over the years resulting to obesity. Have positive thinking overwrite negative self-talk, don't defame yourself rather make positive affirmations concerning your weight and see the miracles.

You will start loving yourself more and therefore work towards that. Positive thinking and meditation are a sure path to enlightenment which when properly practiced lead to inner peace, health, happiness and good interpersonal relationships. Optimists often emerge from difficult situations with less distress, so play safe. Choose to live happier, healthier and don't take life too seriously. There is always some bit of good in everything.

Meditation should have you experience the state of "I am" in an eternal now and stills all else mentally bringing peace. Meditation rejuvenates the body cells and retards decay due to the positive state of mind when all other thoughts are cleared. Positive cell development has often been linked to positive thoughts, leading to cells acquiring energy faster for purposes of growth and repair.

Meditation contributes to spiritual strength, intuitive knowledge by calming the mind and enabling one to attain a state of bliss where the knower, the knowledge and the known mesh into one. Positive thinking and meditation also reinforce the importance of deep and rhythmic breathing to enable the flow of vital energy through the body. Just like no one teaches you to sleep, meditation cannot be taught per se since the ability to shut down lies entirely upon the individual.

All the above combined are the very essence of Yoga exercises for mental, physical and spiritual well-being. So for those out there looking to shed off some of that extra weight, simply follow the 10 days program that seeks to combine all the principles discussed above to maximize on your weight loss. This 10 days program is guaranteed to leave you not only lighter but also healthier and more fit.

The 10 days program will have you adapt to a strict vegan diet together with Yoga exercises that will help you literally transform by losing weight effortlessly for the long term. The weight loss program will have you change your eating habits to cleanse the body of accumulated toxins.

The detox plans should comprise sleeping more, drinking lemon water first thing in the morning, engaging in Yoga exercises, drinking a lot of water and partaking of raw foods which should be properly chewed to help liquefy them. Breath meditations will help you relax and get your mind off cravings.

What's the whole idea behind this 10 days program? It is to take the workload off your bodies organs while helping to improve their performance in and build up on your strength and flexibility. Voila! There you have it! Do you want to improve your digestion, physical appearance, mental clarity, energy and self confidence?

Try out the 10 DAYS program and say goodbye overweight

Chapter 5: The basic principles of Yoga food

Yoga is an ancient spiritual discipline which has been practiced over several centuries. It is a means of calming the mind, and improving health. It is best described as a way of life that embraces several basic principles. Adherence to these will give relief from various ailments and instill a sense of well-being in the individual.

The most well-known aspects of Yoga are yogic exercises and meditation. Yogic diet is less widely discussed but is in fact responsible for many of the benefits of Yoga. Let us find out about the basics of Yoga food and what it entails for health, particularly in relation to weight loss.

What is a yogic food ?:

This type of food is most advised by people practicing Yoga. Yogic food is known as vegetarian food. It can best be described as a food philosophy as envisaged and advocated by Yoga practitioners from time immemorial.

Why do we call it a philosophy?:

This is because the basics of Yoga food involves some principles embraced in following it. What are these principles? Let us examine a few of them:

1. Type of food:

Vegetarianism is the basic principle of the yogic diet. This is based on the surmise that man is basically not carnivorous. Most apes, which are considered predecessors to humans are herbivorous.

The philosophy of not causing unnecessary harm to others may also have played a role in adopting this principle of vegetarianism. Dairy products and nuts are however recommended highly. This provides the precious animal protein required for the body without consuming meat.

2.Quantity of food:

One basic principle of a Yoga diet is that people are advised to eat only half of what they feel is their fill. You can fill a quarter of your stomach with water. One quarter should stay empty for the best digestion results. This helps in keeping the mind and body agile and alert. Never eat until you feel full.

3.Frequency of intake:

According to yogic principles, a person should have at least 3 meals in the day. Start with a light breakfast, after lunch at mid-day and an early supper. All meals are to be equally spaced with a minimum gap of 4 hours between meals.

4.Spices and seasoning:

These are not advocated in a yogic diet. Any food with very strong flavor or a pungent odor is, as a rule, not to be consumed when on a yogic diet. This is because such foods are stimulating in nature and produce more harmful acid in the stomach.

5.Alcohol and stimulating beverages:

Alcohol and stimulating beverages are not allowed for people following a yogic diet. Please never practice Yoga when you are intoxicated or used any type of stimulating product. This not only bad for your body, it is also to avoid injuries.

6.Yogic diet for weight loss:

Yogic diet has a very different approach to the problem of obesity and weight loss. It addresses this problem through a holistic approach. It is not an isolated, concentrated effort, attempting to achieve weight loss by adopting severe and often punishing regimes.

Such attempts can be harmful to the body and results are often temporary.

Yogic foods, on the other hand encourage and inculcate a sense of inner peace and happiness and eliminate the stress imposed by society.

7.Components of yogic diet:

It is a vegetarian diet, chiefly consisting of the following components:

- Whole grains.
- Fresh fruits.
- Raw vegetables.
- Nuts.
- Legumes
- Milk products.

The actual diet advised may vary depending on various factors, like lifestyle, level of physical activity, climate and so on. But the principle remains essentially the same.

8.Role of herbs:

There are several herbs recognized in yogic diet as producing heat in the body. For example ginger, dandelion, turmeric and many more. These may be added to diet to boost metabolism and enhance weight loss.

9.Mindful eating:

By treating eating as a spiritual exercise, you eat only as much as your body needs and no more. On the other hand, if you are eating while watching TV, your mind is not on what you are eating, but on the show on TV. As a result, you are not aware of what you are eating and tend to overeat.

10.Having the right mindset:

The mind is the starting point for effective weight loss. In Yoga, the mind, body, breath and internal organs are all brought into alignment, which makes it easier to achieve weight loss.

11.Yoga exercises:

Various asanas or yogic poses help to lose weight by relaxing the mind while at the same time, exercising the body. The weight of the body itself is used to form stronger muscles and a healthier body. Weight loss is a welcome by-product of adopting a yogic way of life.

We have learned so far about the basics of Yoga food and how it can help you with battling your weight issues in a holistic way. Yogic foods also have the advantage of leaving you more satisfied after the meal with increased satiety. Moreover, by inducing a sense of inner happiness, it will curb your cravings for comfort foods, further helping your weight loss efforts.

A more detailed meal plan can also be discussed keeping specific weight loss goals in mind. Please check out the website www.yogalatinos.com for more information or explain your problems in the contact form on the website.

Chapter 6: What are calories?

I'm sure many of us have come across the term "calories" while reading health and fitness articles, seeking to find out how best to lose weight a couple of times. But what exactly are calories? How are they measured? Let's find out more.

Simply put, a calorie is a unit of energy. To bring the concept closer home, calories are the energy you consume whenever you drink or eat. So why is it important to learn about calories and how they are measured in helping you to lose 10 pounds in 10 days?

The human requires these calories to survive for, without them, our bodies would wither away. It is therefore important to know the right amount of calories needed by our bodies on a daily basis.

How are calories significant in your quest for weight loss? Weight gain comes about as a result of eating too many calories and not burning enough of them through normal body functions such as digestion, breathing, growth and repair of cells. This is why it is good to know how to measure the calorie content of various kinds of food.

When it comes to counting calories for weight loss, it's all a balancing act to between cutting down your calorie intake or burning them out through body processes to achieve your weight loss goals. A combination of both would actually work best.

Calories are provided by carbohydrates, proteins and fat. Fats have the highest concentration of calories. 1 gram of fat contains 9 calories. For carbohydrates and proteins, each gram contains 4 calories. You need to realize that with different body sizes, age, height, gender, physical activity and general state of health comes varying calorie requirements.

Therefore we cannot say that a 60 year old female librarian requires the same number of calories as a 23 year old male rugby player. This is due to the varying metabolic rates. Metabolism is the process by which the body converts the food we eat into energy. This process combines the oxygen we breathe in with the calories in the food and drinks we take in to produce energy.

Men tend to have higher metabolic rates than women of their age and weight due to the fact that they have more muscles in their bodies therefore making men require more calories than women. Also, a person with a larger body size means they have more muscles, meaning they burn more calories. The older a person gets, the more their metabolic rate slows down due to reduced muscle content in the body. These variations are brought about by differing basic metabolic rates which accounts for a large amount of the calories we take in.

How then can the remaining calories be accounted for? The remaining calories are used during food processing and general physical activities that the body engages in such as walking and running. To lose weight therefore, you need to create an energy deficit by taking in fewer calories or by increasing the number of calories you burn through physical activity or doing both at the same time. This principle is what is adopted in the 10 pounds Yoga weight loss in just 10 days!

You are required to determine a safe daily calorie deficit that is pertinent to your metabolic rate, age, sex and level of physical activity. This will determine the food portions you will be taking to aid in your weight loss. Because 3,500 calories are equivalent to one pound of fat, you will need to burn that very same amount of calories in a day to ensure you lose a pound of fat each day for the 10 days. This should mean that your calorie intake should reduce by getting rid of empty calories and eating a healthier set of foods in smaller portions while exercising as often as possible.

To keep track of your progress, it will be important that you keep a weight loss journal to keep track of what you eat together with the calorie content. Account for every calorie you take in by being very keen with your food portions. You should also measure the amount of calories you have burned using a calorie counter to see whether you are headed in the right direction and if not make the necessary adjustments. This could be a great help to get you motivated.

Eat low calorie healthy foods that fill you up such as vegetables and proteins and avoid dressings on your salad as they come loaded with extra calories. Stick to foods such as beans, spinach, lentils and lettuce. Proteins will be important for keeping you full to prevent needless snacking, to boost burning of calories since they require more energy to digest and prevention of muscle loss as a result of calorie deficit.

Maintain a diet that is low on sugar, fat, salt and carbohydrate. Carbohydrates should be avoided because they bind to more water than protein or fats thus contributing to overall body weight through the increased water weight.

Ease in to the diet slowly to avoid shocking your body at once especially when it comes to elimination of carbohydrates. You should also drink a lot of water to replenish fluids lost during exercise and to help keep the stomach full to prevent snacking in between meals. Slight dehydration tends to reduce metabolism and performance of aerobic activities by the body.

It would also be helpful to partner up with other individuals on a similar weight loss journey as you to help boost each other's morale by sticking to similar diets or even working out together. This would also help encourage your weight loss efforts through sharing progress reports with each other for mutual support.

The 10 days weight loss program encourages you to be actively engaged in Yoga exercises that tend to lengthen and strengthen muscles as well as boost aerobic activities of the body through rapid movements thus burning more calories. In order to shed those 10 pounds, you'll need to burn more calories than you consume. Yoga exercises tend to boost proper muscle development meaning boosted metabolic rates.

Engage more in active forms of Yoga to build on your strength through muscle development and cardio, inspired on Yoga workout exercises to support weight loss. Yoga breathing exercises that require long and rhythmic breathing will increase your body's uptake of oxygen that will be used up to break down more calories during exercise. You can supplement the Yoga exercises and diet with aerobic exercises or other sports, such as running, swimming and other active sports to help in burning additional calories.

When it comes to weight loss, a lifestyle change is of key importance. Changing your eating habits has a lot to do with it. Therefore, avoid fad diets and juice cleanses that tend to shock your body. Rather, try losing 10 pounds in 10 days using Yoga and rapidly burn that fat the healthy way.

Try it out today!

Chapter 7: What before the 10 DAYS program?

Before you start with the 10 days program there are some things you need to be aware of. In order to succeed it is important to understand the basics of the program.

Practicing Yoga regularly can influence your weight loss. You now know that Yoga weight loss occurs when a person's calorie intake, that's eating of food or drinking drinks, is less than their caloric usage like energy used daily in exercises. In order to lose weight, one must go through the Yoga practices. To reduce the required weight in 10 days, follow the steps below.

First you should know how many calories you want to lose. You now know that one pound equals to 3500 calories, in order to lose 10 pounds, mathematically, calories of up to 35000 in 10 days should be lost. It's a high value though by following the steps below you will sail through this successfully with no harmful effects to your body normal functioning.

Let's break the 10 days into four equal stages:

Stage One:

Set your objective:

That is to lose 3500 calories per day. You need to reduce your calorie content in your meals, in order to lose a pound each day. You therefore need to know the quantity you should take each day so that you can subtract the 3500 calories daily. To know how many calories you take daily consult a medical professional or check the information that comes included with the food purchased. While you have known the calories you take daily, subtract the 3500, then u have your working figure.

Have records of what you eat:

Have a notebook where you record the food you eat and the calories you are losing. This helps you identify where a challenge is and keep track of how you are going through the exercise. This will tell you if u what to do the next day, like if you should increase what you did previously or reduce or even maintain. This will help you write a work schedule on what you should stick on doing.

Eliminate what is hindering you to your success:

Since you have a good layout plan, avoid junk food that will make the process unsuccessful. Sacrifice what you don't need and throw it away in this 10 days plan. Follow all the simple steps serious, even if you love eating or doing what will make you not lose weight during that period. You have no option, put it away, sacrifice and do not eat them.

Stage two:

Follow healthy eating habits:

Often eat and in small quantities. This will make you eat less and get satisfied too. This keeps you track in following the procedure well and good. While eating often, you should eat slowly so that you don't get false impression that you are full yet you are not. Do not do other things as you also eat. Just keep focused on what you are doing.

Have some knowledge on calorie movement:

Higher calorie per day aid in reducing hour weight, restricting your body causes the body metabolism to slow down and this gives the body an opportunity to get attached to the nutrients for a sweet life.

Avoid stress and have maximum sleep:

When one is on stress he or she is bound to eating more, this is known by research. Therefore this might hinder one from reducing the calorie level. The best way to go is to have enough sleep and to practice Yoga. Yoga burns the calorie level in the body. Sleeping enough makes the body metabolism work well and achieve better under stress.

Consume drinks that is going to make you lose weight:

Carefully look on fat diets and you will realize that by drinking water, lemonade and Sriracha for ten days, it will help you lose weight significantly. Do not drink soda or any other chemical drinks that maintain a lot of sugars and calories.

Be aware that through history water has always been the most important to drink. Water is the most natural to drink, and it does not have bad nutrition.

Stage three:

Always take water:

This fills you up and makes you consume little. Water also keeps your body and organs strong, healthy and hydrated.

Eat vegetables:

Going green helps you lose weight conveniently and faster. The following are the best green vegetables that will help you lose weight : Kale, spinach, cabbage, lettuce and Brussels sprouts.

Avoid processed white food:

Processed food means less or no fiber hence, not a lot nutrients is found in them. The body requires carbs that are not available in processed food like white bread. You need therefore to avoid them during the ten days plan.

Avoid unhealthy fatty foods:

Fatty unhealthy foods aren't good for good health, they make you gain more weight and even become obese. One undergoing this should avoid in order to reduce weight. Even though so one needs to know where to get healthy fats from. They can be achieved by eating low-fat dairy products. One should also reduce sodium intake and eating at night. Eating at night is unhealthy, also people end up eating unhealthy food with high fats.

Stage four:

Do regular exercises daily:

Going for gym has been proved to be healthy especially when one needs to lose weight. This helps to burn up excess fats in the body as exercising makes our body parts active. Other exercising activities includes: dancing, football, cricket, netball, walking, cleaning (your room), hiking and of course doing Yoga.

Switch to Yoga training and do it always:

Create a weight lose lifestyle with Yoga. Follow the tips and hints that you took note of by reading this book. Implement the Yoga exercises to your new way of life. Keep doing what you learned regularly during the 10 days plan, plus the time after, and success is on your way.

Chapter 8: Introduction to the 10 DAYS program

The program is made to fit in the full planned schedules that people have these days. When you don't have time to practice one hour a day, or eat in seven or eight portions a day, this program will fit perfect for you. The 10 days program will ask you to do every day exercises for about fifteen minutes. Even though your free time is short, this program can fit just in.

Even after reaching that dream number on the weighing scale, one needs to continue on the journey to a healthy lifestyle. In the days to come follow these 5 simple guiding principles and you will never have to fear the weighing scale again.

1. Eat as much food that fits into both your palms because that's exactly how much your stomach is built to digest at a time.
2. Break your meals down into small portions eating at least three times a day. Perfectly would be to eat seven to eight times a day.
3. Drink at least 1.5 liters of water every day, if you can, drink up to 3.5 liters a day. However, avoid water intake half an hour before and after meals as it can lead to indigestion and acidity.

4. While eating your main meals sip on a cup of hot green tea which is a natural diuretic and aids digestion. If you don't enjoy tea then do the same with warm water.

5. Yoga keeps you young, an although the program is based on fifteen minutes of exercises, you can increase the time to half an hour everyday along with a fifteen minute walk to get maximum result.

   This is one punch that keeps us healthy and our families happy.

Going trough each day, shall allow you to eat three times or more if possible. You will not have a low energy status or have bad feelings, because you follow this diet. No, by following this program you will have more energy and you will feel better than ever before.

Are you ready for the 10 days program? START TODAY!

The 10 DAYS program: Day one

Now that you have decided that you want to have a healthier lifestyle, here are the instructions for how you can get started. Day one is the first day of the program and it is very important to start the day, and your path to a new you, right.

If you have already tried crash diets and "wonder plans" before, you know that focusing only on what you eat is not enough. The results don't show, or don't last. It's frustrating and a period of deprivation, where you stop yourself from having what you really want, is followed by binge-eating and overeating on food that's just not good for you. And you can't even enjoy that, because you feel guilty about ruining your diet.

Yoga, with it's combined plan of diet and exercise, is a long-term, balanced solution where you can eat well, enjoy yourself, and also feel happier and more centered. This is a description of what you can do on your first day, both in terms of exercise and diet. Follow this plan and you can relax, challenge yourself, and also enjoy yourself as you start on the journey to rediscovering yourself.

Since this is your first day, start slowly. Get to know where your body is and what it needs. Before you even begin, make sure that you are in the right environment for you to relax. It would be best if you could go outdoors and lay your mat out on some grass in a park. If there is some water nearby, that would give you some positive energy and the sound of moving water can be very soothing and calming. If it is early in the morning, which is ideal, place your mat facing the rising sun. If it's already quite warm, you can also do this in the shade.

In case there is no appropriate place outdoors, you can also do Yoga at home. Find a clean and quiet place to relax and lay down your mat. You can play some Buddhist hymns, nature sounds or other music as something soothing in the background.

Sit down on your Yoga mat and cross your legs. Tuck them into "Padmasana" (Lotus Pose) if you can. If that is difficult, just sit with your legs crossed and with your feet on top of each other. Like other exercise, it is important to push yourself, but in Yoga it is also very important to know your body and let it relax into positions. Don't push yourself more than is comfortable, because that puts you at risk for injury.

Once you are sitting comfortably, with your legs crossed, move your thighs a little with your hands, adjusting them to feel as comfortable as possible. Sit with your back straight (don't slouch) and face facing forward.

If you are facing the sun, feel the warm energy on your skin, entering your body, waking you up and giving you strength. Take a few minutes to meditate on your intentions that you have made about the decision to make a lifestyle choice. Sometimes it will be difficult. Make a promise to yourself to try it out for at least this 10 days, to see what kind of changes it brings and how it makes you feel.

The main exercise for today focuses on a major area of concern for most people, the belly. While sitting in the Padmasana or Cross Legged Position, push your belly sharply in and breathe out. Repeat. As you push the belly in, the air will be pushed out of your lungs. When you relax, air will automatically fill back in. Repeat pushing in the belly and pushing out air, with one push per second, for as long as you can keep doing it. Try to do it for at least three minutes. Then rest. And then repeat for three more minutes.

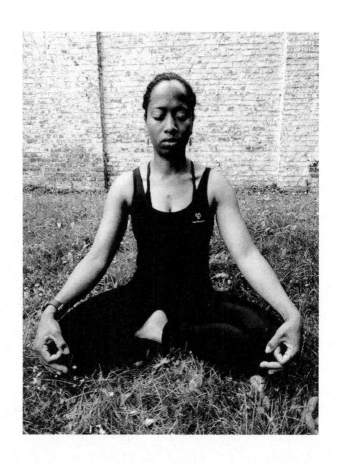

After you have done this Pranayam (breathing exercise),
take a short rest before doing the second exercise of the day.
Stand up, with your feet next to each other and your body
straight. Lift your arms and bring your hands down in front
of your feet. Bend your knees now if you have to. Walk, step
or jump back, until your feet are now away from your hands
and your body forms a triangle with the ground, the ground

being the bottom line, your arms up to hips being a second line and your legs being the third. This is the down dog position. Hold for five breaths before coming back to an upright position. Do this three times.

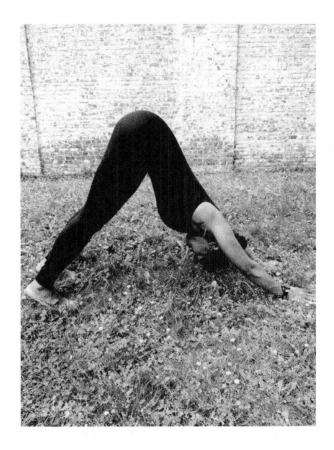

Namaste, your fifteen minutes of Yoga routine for today has now ended. You already finished the exercises for day one.

In addition to exercise, diet is also important. Here is a suggestion for your first day. Start your morning with a glass of cool, plain water. We put lots of toxins into our body throughout the day and your body needs clean water to flush it out.

After your fifteen minute routine, have breakfast. Have a low-fat, fresh vegetarian meal. Low sugar muesli or cornflakes with milk, yogurt or cottage cheese is a good idea. You can load it up with fresh fruits or a few mixed nuts (make sure they are unsalted!).

After minimum four hours is the lunch. Have a hearty salad with lots of fresh, leafy vegetables for lunch. You can add a few nuts and a spoonful of virgin olive oil with some salt and pepper as dressing, but don't use prepackaged, store-bought dressing. You can have some Pita bread or Chapati with your salad, but make sure the portion size is slightly smaller than you would normally eat.

In case you get hungry between meals, have some fresh fruit as a snack. This will not only fill you up but give you fibers, which are very important for digestion and getting rid of toxins.

After a long day, a healthy dinner is very important. Have some lentil soup or daal (dahl), with turmeric, which helps the body break down fat. Pair this with a bowl of either plan rice or jeera rice, which has a light stir fry of cumin seeds, excellent for digestion.

Remember to drink lots of water through the day and avoid processed food and drinks, especially those with too much salt and sugar.

You was great on the first day!

The 10 DAYS program: Day two

So maybe you've been trying out all the weight loss and diet programs out there and none of them have seemed to work, or maybe some have worked momentarily before the weight slipped right back in. Tasking! Huh? Well I think it's about time you changed tact and embraced the Yoga food and Yoga exercises that make you lose 10 pounds In 10 days. Imagine that!

Yoga exercises together with the proper diet are guaranteed to give you weight loss results within 10 days. In addition to helping in weight reduction, this vegetarian diet helps in detoxifying your body. A point to note is that the Yoga diet should be eased into for beginners, nothing drastic to avoid shocking the body.

We are done with day one and this is day two, so hurrah! You are on the right track. Just keep your eyes fixed on the end goal, keep going with the exercises and diets but please do not despair, for every great journey begins with just but a single step.

As regards Yoga exercises that will aid in weight loss for beginners on day two, they are best done early in the morning and you should work on Yoga exercises that are cardio inspired such as breathing exercises to foster a sensation similar to that gotten from aerobic workouts to boost metabolism. These may include:

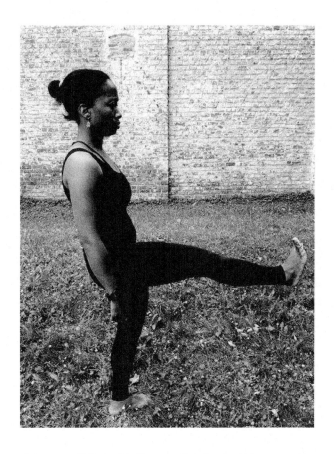

Front stretching and leg circling, which simply requires you to stand straight with your arms raised at a 90 degree angle or holding your femur.

Then start stretching with the right and left leg in alternation while while circling the down part from the leg, counting up to a total of about 20 times. This exercise will be useful in helping to reduce abdominal fat.

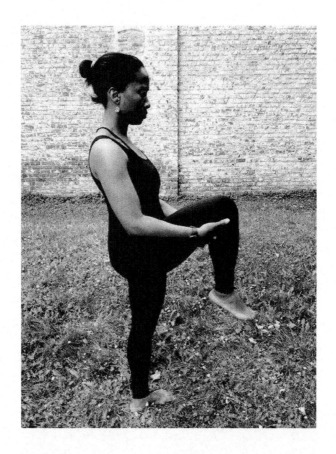

Leg circling is a great way to exercise that helps in reducing thigh and abdominal fat. You simply have to lie down flat on your Yoga mat, then lift one leg, let's say the right leg and circle it in clockwise motion ten times, then circle it in anticlockwise motion ten times. Repeat this for the left leg as well. Then raise both legs and circle them in both clockwise and anticlockwise motion.

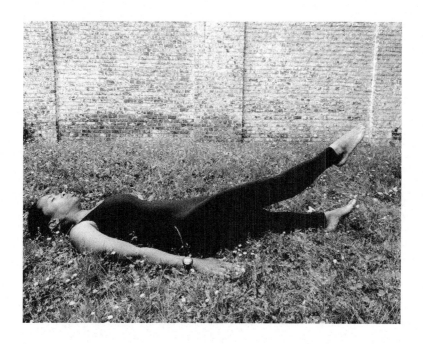

The side bend whereby you lift your arms over your head then bending to the right and maintain that position while counting till ten. Come back to the original position, then bend to the left and count till ten, then come back to the initial standing position. This is a wonderful Yoga exercise that will help in reduction of fat and will also tone your abdominal muscles.

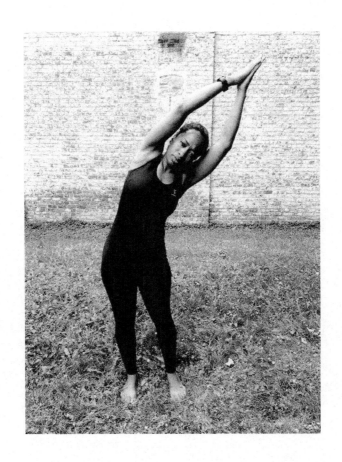

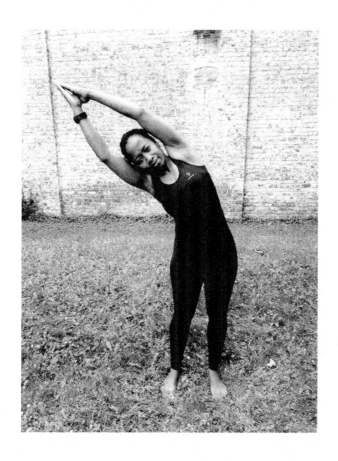

Namaste, your fifteen minutes of Yoga routine for today has now ended. You already finished the exercises for day two.

Here's what day two of your Yoga weight loss menu should consist of.

Upon rising up in the morning, it is important to kick start the day with a glass of warm water. This should be taken 15-30 minutes before taking the actual breakfast to encourage proper digestion by flushing out toxins in the digestive tract.

Lemon water will also help in fighting hunger cravings that you might encounter in the course of the day. Please ensure that you drink about 10 to 12 glasses of water throughout the day to keep your metabolism up and running and to help prevent snacking.

For breakfast, you may have a bowl of steel cut oats cooked in milk and toss on blueberry or strawberry fruits and nuts. This could be taken together with green tea or a banana smoothie. For the smoothie, throw in a banana, spinach leaves, carrots and unsweetened soya milk and blend them together to be taken before and after carrying out Yoga exercises to complement the diet for weight loss.

Why a banana smoothie? Well, bananas are known to increase metabolism thus are a great boost in weight reduction. Oats have a rich fiber content and will help in burning fat and boost your body's metabolism. Don't skip breakfast to minimize your chances of overindulging in your next meal.

Your lunch meal should be a proper one consisting of salads without any form of dressing, vegetables and a rich protein source. You could have vegetable salad and a small serving of boiled kidney beans seasoned with cayenne pepper to add flavor and boost metabolism. Beans contain fiber which leave you feeling full throughout the day thus promoting weight loss by cutting off incessant eating. Proteins are especially great for weight loss since they take more work to digest meaning they end up burning more calories in order to be metabolized and used.

Dinner should also be high on vegetables and proteins. You could opt for baked or steamed vegetables, a slice of mature cheese and a cup of green herbal tea. Try to have your dinner early enough to give your body ample time to digest everything before going to bed, since metabolism tends to drastically slow down when we are asleep.

So far you are good on day two, always remember that lasting weight loss as is with the 10 days Yoga weight loss program isn't built on food deprivation. Be sure to eat at least three times while concentrating on low calorie foods a day with a healthy snack such as an apple at least once in between, if the hunger pangs persist. Writing down a weight loss journal will also help keep you on track and motivate you to continue.

You will however have to be very diligent with the Yoga exercises since increased physical activity has a very heavy bearing on your body's ability to carry out metabolic activities at optimum level.

Pair up with a fellow friend also seeking to lose a few pounds and share on how day two fared on for both of you and encourage each other to press on. Above all, remember that the weight loss is a personal journey for development so do not despair. The best is yet to come. Press on as you await impressive results for the days to come.

Rest good and you will be ready for tomorrow!

The 10 DAYS program: Day three

Yoga is an ancient discipline whose practice allows to significantly improve both physical and psychological well being. Like other activities focused on breathing, exercises and relaxation techniques, this ancient practice of oriental origin (that is now widespread to the West) has many beneficial effects.

The simple combination of physical movement, breathing exercises, relaxation techniques, and a healthy diet, has brought Yoga to be included among the useful activities not only to improve the physical fitness but also to improve the mental status.

In a research conducted by the Fred Hutchinson Center, it was discovered that Yoga enhances the body awareness, with an increased focus on the feeling of satiety and improves the self-acceptance, which means the increment of personal balance and, therefore, less need to seek compensation eating.

The first phenomenon is particularly important: people often eat too much because they don't realize the feeling of satiety that comes from the stomach or realize it too late. It is exactly the space created between the "need" (bite of hunger) and the reaction that enables us to see clearly what are the constraints and the habits that influence our behavior. Yoga also stimulates awareness of the present moment and that you can learn to enjoy the food instead of eating it mechanically.

Then the relaxation techniques help to relax the body and to eliminate stress and the excessive amount of cortisol in the blood, grafting a mechanism that facilitates weight loss. This means that Yoga therapy for weight loss can be extremely effective, but it requires three essential prerequisites without which you will not see great results.

The requisites are: "patience, constancy and collaboration". This is a slow process, but thanks to this gradual weight loss it keeps the results over time.

If you only diligently follow a few simple rules, but don't change your way of life and your habits, the knowledge developed will soon be forgotten and lost, and the intent will be useless.

Returning to a balanced weight is a delicate and important internal process to which you must dedicate time every day, so cut out a bit of time from your busy schedule and dedicate it to yourself. The best thing to do is to dedicate a certain time for your daily Yoga practice. Make sure all of your electronic devices are turned off or set on silence mode, and it would be best if the other inhabitants of the house are out or busy with other chores in order to not disturb you.

Tell your family or friends how important it is for you to spend that time on Yoga practice and ask to not be interrupted except in the case of emergency. Find a quiet place where to practice Yoga. It is very important to identify a specific space where you feel comfortable and where you can easily do your daily Yoga session.

And now it's time to start the improvement of your lifestyle, reducing stress and body weight. For the third day of Yoga exercise, you will do only the position of the Cobra.
This position will help you make your back more flexible, regulate the digestive system and tone the muscles of the abdomen. Lie down on your back and bend your arms, putting your hand on either side of the chest, with the elbows close to the body.

Start breathing by lifting the head, then the chest and finally the abdomen. The initial bending must be done using only your back muscles, the arms must be used only to maintain balance. Leaving the legs and feet together and tense, slowly stretch out your arms, increasing the curvature of your back. Push your hips down and clench your buttocks. The head is bowed and the eyes are directed upwards, leaving the facial muscles relaxed. Hold the position of the cobra for about 15-20 seconds then relax. Repeat for 5-10 minutes.

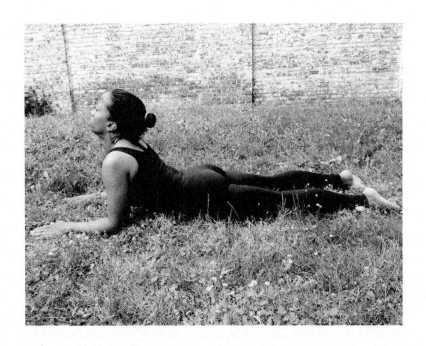

Take a small break from five minutes if you need to recover. Now start over again. Leaving the legs and feet together and tense, stretch out your arms flat by increasing the curvature of the column; push your hips down and clench your buttocks. The head is bowed, and the eyes are directed upwards, leaving the facial muscles relaxed. Hold the position for 15-20 seconds. Repeat for 5-10 minutes.

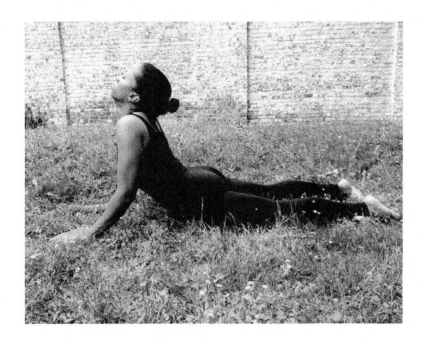

Namaste, your fifteen minutes of Yoga routine for today has now ended. You already finished the exercises for day three.

To achieve the maximum benefit from this splendid Yoga day (and I hope you'll continue with the fourth day), the advice is to also follow a correct augmentation that will help you lose weight in a healthy way.
The delicious menu for the third day is the following.

For breakfast drink a cup of green mint tea with a cup of muesli with nuts or almonds; avoid the fruit for the breakfast and consume it during the day if you get hungry.

At lunchtime, eat raw fennel and about 80 grams of rice noodles with a spoonful of pesto sauce.

Finally, for dinner you can eat 2 potatoes, chicory, and escarole, boiled and seasoned with oil, lemon and a teaspoon of toasted sesame seeds. Besides, 120 grams of low-fat cottage cheese, a whole grain bun or 2 rice cakes. For dessert, a baked apple with a pinch of cinnamon and a teaspoon of honey.

Trust me, following these simple rules, not only life will seem more easy and pleasant, but you will also lose weight gradually and definitive without running the risk of regaining the weight lost.

Keep your head up! You are on the right track!

The 10 DAYS program: Day four

Congratulations on deciding to become a better, happier, and healthier you. Today we will discuss various Yoga exercises that can help you build your body in the right direction you are aiming for. We will also go over a few healthier food decisions you can make throughout your day to help slim your body. Following this guide over the course of just 10 days, can help you shed 10 pounds or more!

 Today you can make it little harder. Repeat both of these exercises twice each, before each meal throughout the course of your day. Make sure to do basic stretches to prepare your body! This first exercise you will be working with will help the back, thighs, hips, and stomach.

The bridge will help strengthen your lower body and core along with lengthening and stretching out your spine. Begin by laying down on your Yoga mat, arms should be alongside your body, palms facing down. You should be bent at the knees with both feet flat on the floor, about hip width apart. Inhale in as you extend your spine off of the ground rolling it into an arch as you push down lightly with your feet.

Extend the chest by walking your shoulders in and pressing down into them, and your arms, for the support your body is looking for. Make sure your hips, buttocks, legs, and spine are all working together to make a slight arch. You may interlace your fingers together and hold them underneath the buttocks if it will give you a better balance.

Hold this pose for about four to eight breaths until you exhale and roll the spine slowly back onto your mat. Repeat this same Yoga exercise four to five times. When needed you may also use a Yoga block under your hips to help support your weight.

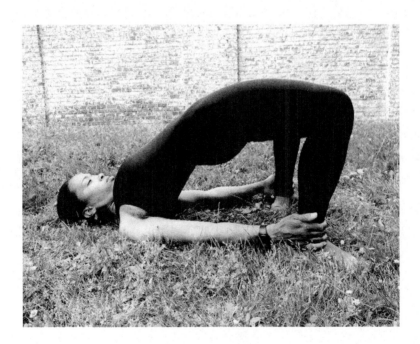

The half spinal twist is going to be your second exercise for today. It helps with opening up the lungs for a better air way passage. It helps to stimulate the digestive system which heavily aides in weight loss. It also assists with toning of the thighs.

Begin with sitting, legs stretched in front of you and feet together. Now bend your right leg, bring your right heel as it is bent at the knee, over beside the left hip. You have the option to keep the left leg straight or you can bend it and bring the foot close to your buttocks. Now raise the right arm up and then around the upright knee to entwine them as you put the left hand directly behind you. Slowly twist at the waist as you look over your right shoulder.

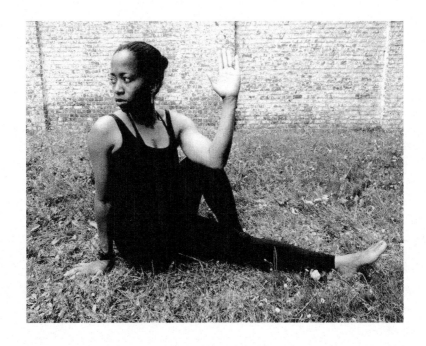

You should feel a nice gentle stretch throughout your body, hold and continue this for a few long breaths. Slowly return to the starting position. Repeat this Yoga exercise with the opposite leg and arms.

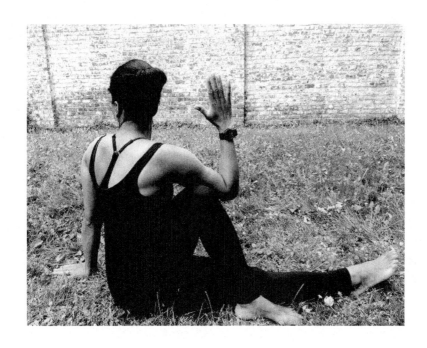

Namaste, your fifteen minutes of Yoga routine for today has now ended. You already finished the exercises for day four.

Oatmeal is the best way to start off your day, it is a whole grain powerhouse! Not only does every serving of oatmeal supply you with a heart healthy source of fiber, it is also high in carbohydrates and is a rich source of protein. Packed with calcium and potassium, oatmeal is never the wrong answer and can aide in healthy weight loss as well. 1 cup of low fat milk to ever 1/2 serving size of oatmeal will do the trick! Add a hand full of blue berries or what ever fruit you are in the mood for and enjoy!

Lunch time is just as important as breakfast! For lunch try opting in a real banana strawberry smoothie. Put 1 banana and about 5 strawberries into a blender followed by 1/4th a cup of non fat milk. Do not forget 3 tablespoons of plain fat free yogurt! Add in 6 to 7 ice cubes and blend until you find a consistency suited for you.

Along with the smooth, enjoy a nice green bean salad consisting of 1 pound of slim green beans, 1 cup of crumbled feta cheese, and 1 cup of sliced tomatoes. Even add onions for extra flavor if you like! Follow that with 2 tablespoons of oil, a little red wine vinegar, and almonds for added flavor. You can always tweak it to your liking with some garlic.

Tofu quinoa stir fry is a great option for dinner. Prepare 1 1/3 cups of uncooked quinoa with 1/2 pound of firm tofu, spice it up with some garlic and herbs if you desire. Add in a table spoon of soya sauce along with your favorite vegetables such as broccoli and pepper medleys and you will have a delicious, filling, yet very healthy dinner ahead of you.

You have the right spirit to continue!

The 10 DAYS program: Day five

Half Way There! Congratulations on making it to day five of the 10 days program! I am sure you can already start to see the hard work paying off! Let's start off another awesome day with a fifteen minute Yoga session. Below are the exercises you will be doing today. Today is a little different. You can choose to do four out of seven exercises from below.

Before we begin, one small piece of advice: Go easy on yourself. If you find a pose too hard to do, break it down and do only parts of it. Yoga is not about wriggling your way into crazy poses, it is about feeling good in your way of life.

- Anjali Mudra

Start by sitting on the mat cross legged. Now, bring your hands together at the palms with the fingers pointed upwards. They should be positioned in front of your heart. Take 15 deep, slow breathes. This pose is excellent for entering into a meditative state of mind.

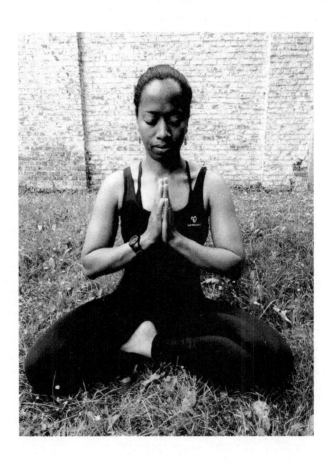

- Bound Angle Pose (Baddha Konasana)

Stretch your feet in front of you. Now bring the soles of the feet together and as close to the pelvis as possible. Try to drop your feet towards the floor. It's OK, if your knees don't touch the floor in the beginning. If you feel your hips are too tight, try sitting on top of a pillow or a blanket instead of the mat. This will help improve posture and also open up the hips.

Now, hold the big toes of your feet with the first two fingers and press the feet firmly together as well as onto the floor. Hold this position for ten breaths. This pose provides a good stretch to the inner thigh and groins and also helps in opening up and improving the flexibility of the hips.

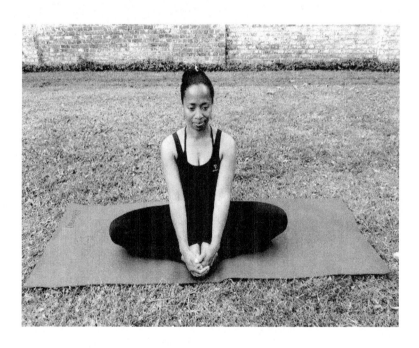

- Blossoming Lotus Pose (VikasitaKamalaana)

Sit upright on the mat with the soles of the feet touching each other, relax your knees. Put your hand underneath your calves such that the calves are resting on your hands and the hands are touching the ground. Inhale, tighten your abs and lift your legs upwards while balancing yourself on your tailbone.

The head, chest and the spine should be straight. Hold the pose for five breathes before returning to original position. Repeat ten times. In case you are having difficulties balancing yourself, use a wall for the first few times. This pose is beneficial for your abs, hips and thighs and also improves your balance and coordination skills.

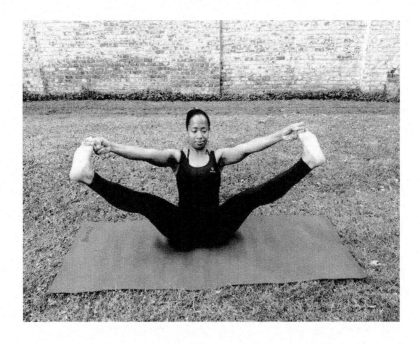

- Downward Facing Dog (Adho Mukha Svanasana)

Start by coming on your hands and knees. The hands should be parallel to each other the shoulder should come above the wrists and the hips above the knees (This pose is called the Table Pose). Now, exhale and lift your knees off the floor and push your hip up towards the ceiling in a smooth, gliding motion.

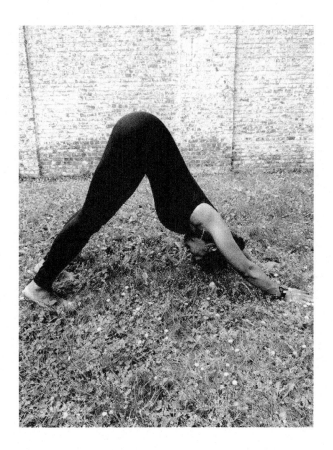

Try to keep the knees straight if you can. After holding the pose for 1-2 seconds, inhale and slowly come back to the kneeling position.

Repeat for eight breaths. This pose helps improve blood circulation and also reduces anxiety and tension.

- Upward Facing Dog (Urdhva Mukha Svanasana)

As before, start by coming in the table pose. The hands should be parallel to each other, the shoulder should come above the wrists and the hips above the knees. Now, slowly drop the hips toward the floor such that the thigh, knee and feet are touching the floor and are stretched straight.

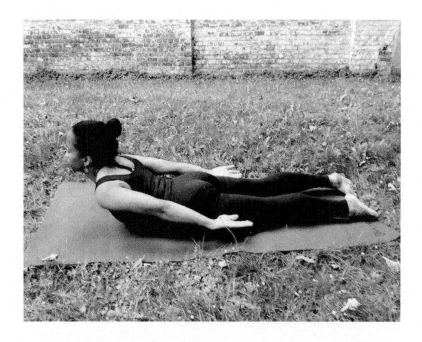

The top of the feet should also touch the floor. Inhale and press the palms down, push the shoulder blades against each other and press the chest forward.

Hold the pose for five breathes and then bent the knees and bring the hip back up to the starting position.

- Locust pose (Shalabhasana)

Start by lying on your stomach with the arms at the sides. Bring your hands underneath the thighs to support them. Now, inhale and slowly bring your legs, shoulders and head upwards.

Hold the pose for one second before exhaling and returning to the original position. Repeat for ten breathes. If you find it difficult to do the pose, first start by lifting one leg and then the other and slowly progress until you master it. This pose stretches and strengthens the muscles of the spine, butt, back and thighs.

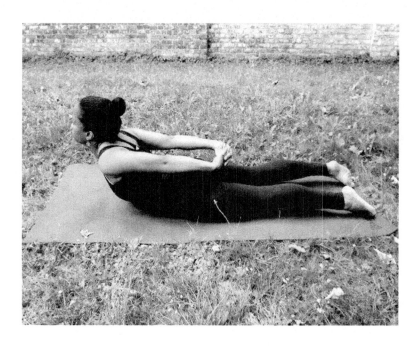

- Corpse Pose (Shavasana)

Lie flat on your back with feet placed slightly apart. Place your arms slightly spread apart from your body. Take slow, deep breathes and bring your focus to all the different parts of the body.

Starting with your right leg, the right knee, moving on to the left leg and so on. Stay in the pose for around 15-20 breathes. This pose helps the body to go into a deep, meditative state of rest, thereby relieving stress.

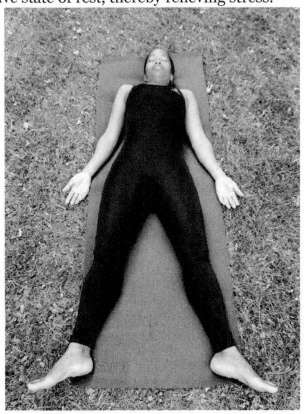

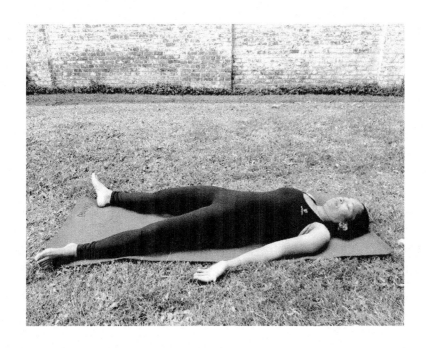

Namaste, your fifteen minutes of Yoga routine for today has now ended. You already finished the exercises for day five. Now let's move on to the diet part of our weight loss mission.

Breakfast is the most important meal in Yoga. Start by having a hydrating beverage at least thirty minutes prior to breakfast. Green tea, lemon in lukewarm water or even fresh natural water is good enough. After the drink, have a bowl of porridge to ensure fiber intake. Grains used in the porridge can be oats, quinoa, barley, etc. Porridge also has the added benefit of being a very good source of energy that will keep you going till lunch.

According to Yoga, lunch is also an important meal of the day. This is because the body's ability to make use of sugar in the food is maximum at noon. Again, start with an early glass of water. Follow it up with a large green salad consisting of ample green leaves. Ingredients can include arugula, endive, radicchio, tomato, bell pepper, lettuce, etc. Key is to maximize the content of greens. Finish the meal with a veggie burger if you are really hungry.

Go light for dinner. Start with a soup, say, cream of mushroom or cream of basil, have some beans with a 3/4 cup of brown rice and finish off with a green juice. Post dinner snacks are a strict no-no.

Now, hit the bed early and get ample sleep before you begin day six of your weight loss journey.

Note: You might be wondering what to do after the 10 days program. You might have had difficulties perfecting certain poses during your sessions. You can work on improving them. The poses being taught in this program are the basic one. Once you master them, your body will be flexible enough to move onto the advanced poses. Sites like www.yogalatinos.com provide a lot of poses with clear instructions.

However, As I said earlier, Yoga is a way of life. It does not end with you mastering numerous poses; it has to be integrated into your daily routine to help you live a healthy, meaningful life.

Good work! You are half way!

The 10 DAYS program: Day six

Starting out your day feeling good is the key to have a wonderful day. In order to feel good you need to do your body good. Practicing Yoga daily and eating a well balanced vegetarian diet, is an excellent way to live.

There are many Yoga poses that are extremely easy and relaxing. When you are new to Yoga you do not want to jump into something to difficult that will end up causing damage to your body. A very relaxing Yoga pose is the garland and intense side stretch. Both poses flow together with ease, and can be modified for your skill level.

To begin, stand with your feet wider apart than your hips, and slightly pointed outwards. Bend your knees until your bottom is about two inches from the floor, squeezing your calves and your thighs. Inhale and exhale. Now bring your arms into your chest into the prayer position in front of your heart. Inhale deeply and exhale slowly. Open your knees and stay in this position for thirty seconds to one minute.

Continue to inhale and exhale. Now push your bottom up into standing position and exhale. While inhaling continue with hands in prayer position and push up to the sky lengthening your spine. Bring arms down to sides while exhaling. You have completed the garland.

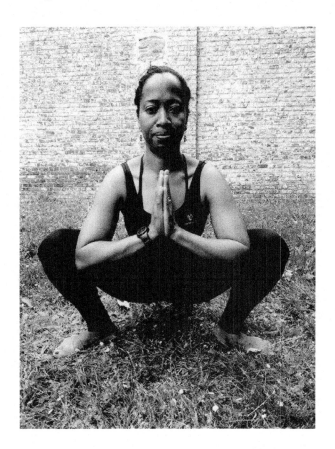

Now you will begin the intense side stretch. In the same position as you have ended the garland in, you will inhale and step back with your left foot about five inches. As you bend forward as if your waist is a hinge, exhale. Only bend to where you feel comfortable, the goal is to meet your chin with your shin. In this position breath deeply five times. Inhale as you lift your upper body back to the beginning position. Switch legs and repeat. You will feel especially energized after completely the garland and intense side stretch pose.

These poses will help to lengthen your spine, while stretching out your legs and arms. The poses will burn enough calories so that you will not feel over worked or burnt out. You will feel at peace in the prayer pose as you breath deeply. Getting plenty of protein is extremely important for individuals wanting to master Yoga. Yoga does your body a lot of good. It helps with flexibility, strength, and toning your body. On the inside of your body it is helping with circulation and balances your metabolism. The most important benefit of Yoga is relieving stress. As you do each pose, try to think of a place that you feel most safe and free from problems.

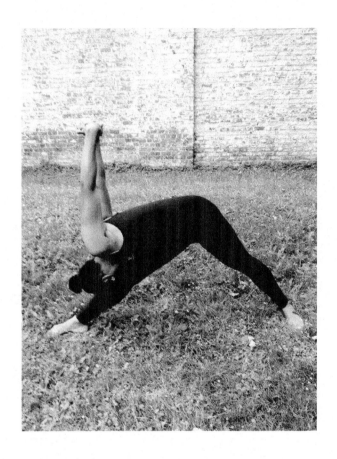

Namaste, your fifteen minutes of Yoga routine for today has now ended. You already finished the exercises for day six.

Now you should be ready for breakfast, since Yoga is best done on an empty stomach. You will be ready for a full day of healthy energizing Yoga food. These meals are super easy to make and completely vegetarian. All three of these meals are low calorie to ensure your goal of losing 10 pounds in 10 days. You will find them extremely delicious, while keeping you full and focused for your busy day. After enjoying them you will not even realize you are eating to lose weight.

For breakfast enjoy a vegetarian breakfast burrito. Load a warmed tortilla full avocado, and a half a cup of black beans for some muscle building protein. To spice up the flavor add in a pinch of paprika. Sprinkle over the top some lemon juice. Lemon juice is scientifically proven to support weight loss.

For a super easy lunch, enjoy a veggie soup. You can use any type of bread you want, and top it with cucumbers, lettuce, tomato, green peppers, and onions. It is also nice to add Dijon mustard for a little extra flavor. This lunch is perfect for the middle of the day, because it is so quick and easy to make and have low calories.

To end your day on a good note, with a satisfying dinner try some vegetarian linguine. This recipe is great because you really can do anything you want with it. After boiling the linguine noodles, the choices of toppings are endless. Try different veggie combos, like crunchy red peppers or zucchini, these are great choices to keep you full and satisfied. Then to tie all the flavor together add some olive oil and Parmesan cheese.

All three of these meals are low calorie, and guaranteed to keep you full. They also taste great, so you will enjoy eating. By the end of day six you will feel great and are over half way through your diet. Losing 10 pounds in 10 days will be easier than you ever dreamed. By the end of the 10 days, not only will you look good but you will definitely feel good!

You will never give up!

The 10 DAYS program: Day seven

As you have probably understood until the seventh day of the diet, Yoga can help you lose weight and get in shape. The particular positions of Yoga are capable of reactivating the metabolism and, especially, to strengthen the muscles of the body.

Another great characteristic of Yoga is that also acting on the mind, relaxing it and reducing the stress-related phenomena, such as emotional eating, which has a negative impact on the health. In addition, this important benefit, Yoga practice, will make your body much more elastic, toned and flexible. Of course, keep in mind that this good practice must always be associated with a healthy lifestyle and a balanced diet to be truly effective.

For the seventh day of the program, we're proposing two simple exercises to start the day, one that will have benefits mainly on your internal organs, and the second that will help you remove the fat from your abdomen and not only there.

Begin your day with the Sage Marichi's pose. This simple pose will stimulate your digestion and removes the toxins from the internal organs. This pose also strengthens and lengthens your spine, helping you become more flexible and relaxed. So let's see how to do it.

From a seated position with the legs stretched forward and the feet close together, bend the right knee bringing the heel near the buttocks and keep your left leg stretched. Both hands are on the ground. Now, stretching the spine, relax your shoulders and keep your buttocks in contact with the floor. Exhale and begin to rotate your torso to the right knee, lean the left hand behind and turn the head to the right.

At each exhalation increase the twisting and lean the back of your right elbow on the outside of your right knee. Hold the position for thirty seconds up to one minute and slowly repeat the position on the other side. Pay attention not to bring your shoulders toward your ears and do not bend the spine. Repeat the position for 7-8 times.

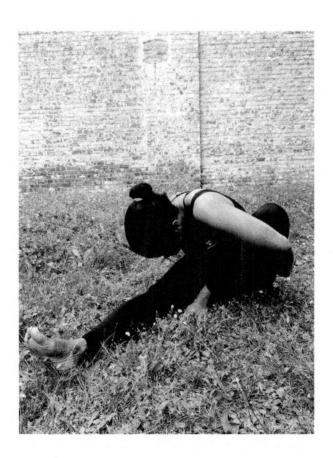

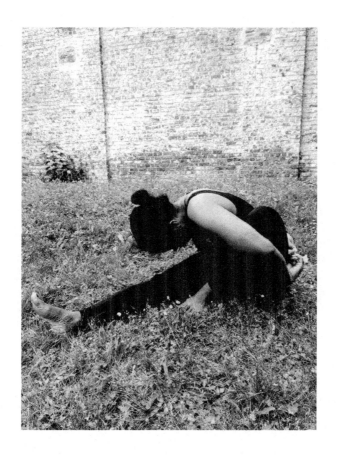

Now, that you are definitely more relaxed, it's time to practice the second Yoga position, the Boat pose. This position will help you reduce the fat localized on the abdomen and thighs, strengthening the abdomen and hip flexure, and will also strengthen your balance and the lumbar sacral spine. In addition, it can alleviate gastric distress, stimulate kidney, thyroid and bowel.

For this pose, sit on the floor with your legs straight forward and your torso perpendicular to the ground. Breathe deeply several times, keep the spine straight, bend your knees, lift your feet and lean backward causing the thighs to form an angle of about 45 degrees with the floor. Keep the hands on the ground, close to your sides, with your fingers pointing toward your feet.

After finding the balance, slowly straighten your knees, bringing the tip of the toes just above eye level. The angle should be of about 90 degrees. Now raise your arms straight, until they are parallel to the floor, with the hands close to the knees. Spread the shoulder blades and stretch starting from the fingers.

Breathe normally. Slightly bent the chin toward the sternum; in this way, the base of the skull raises. Hold this position for ten to twenty seconds. Melt the legs with an exhalation and relax. Repeat this position for about seven minutes.

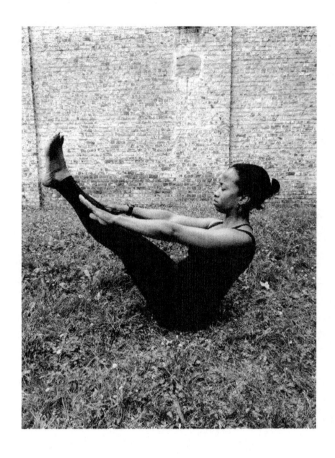

Namaste, your fifteen minutes of Yoga routine for today has now ended. You already finished the exercises for day seven.

Of course, to really get the most benefit in terms of stress reduction and especially in terms of body weight loss, add to the seventh day of your diet this tasty menu.

Start your day with a delicious breakfast consisting in a centrifuged of fruit and vegetables with two tablespoons of muesli, one slice of whole grain bread spread with honey and a cup of barley coffee. If you get hungry until lunch, eat a fresh fruit, but pay attention to get a season fruit, possibly of organic production.

For lunch, prepare a dish of quinoa with fresh veggies. All you have to do is boil about 80 grams of quinoa and season it with 100 grams of steamed mixed vegetables and steamed Brussels sprouts. If you need a snack until supper, a white yogurt is a great choice.

For dinner, prepare a delicious cream soup with 70 grams of boiled peas and flavor it with extra virgin olive oil and a teaspoon of Parmesan cheese. For the main course, choose a mixed salad topped with a spoonful of yogurt sauce, a whole grain bun or two rice cakes.

As you may have noticed there is nothing stressing or tiresome. If you follow with perseverance the Yoga style, you will definitely reach great results in terms of both weight loss and health gain, but remember: it takes discipline and perseverance.

You are on the road to success!

The 10 DAYS program: Day eight

You've made it to day eight of the 10 days program. Take a second to congratulate yourself for making it this far. Most people claim it's too hard and give up on the first days, but NOT YOU! You're a warrior and you're committed to your goal of losing that extra ten pounds. Any yogi would be proud of you. Now, let's start the day with some Yoga.

Triangle Pose:
Stand with your feet together. Raise your hands up above your head and interlock your fingers. Lift your right foot and take a big step to the side at least four feet. Brings your arms down to the side and keep your hands at shoulder height, stretching in opposite directions.

Now for the hard part. Turn your right foot to point in the same direction as your right hand and keep your left foot solid on the ground, pointing forward. Bend your right knee until your thigh bone is parallel to the ground and lean into it, keeping both feet in one line. Lock both knees and shift your body weight to your right foot. Twist your body from the waist, moving both arms at the same time until your right elbow is inside your right knee and your left arm is pointing up to sky.

Touch your chin to your left shoulder. Point your right fingers in between your toes and make sure that they are not touching the ground. Push your right knee out from the inside with your elbow. Hold here for fifteen seconds then reverse out of the pose, coming out the exact opposite way that you went in. Repeat the pose but this time bend into your left knee. This pose is good for strengthening the muscles of your pelvic floor as well your thighs.

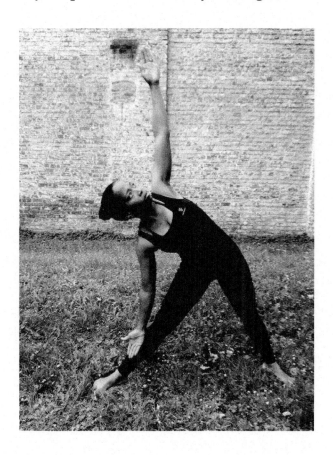

Standing Separate Leg Head To Knee Pose:

Stand with your heels and toes together and take a two-foot step to the right. Turn your right foot 90 degrees clockwise and your left foot 45 degrees in. Face the right and twist your hips so that they are aligned. Raise both arms high above your head, tuck your chin to your chest and bend forward from the waist until your head touches your right knee.

Bend your right knee if you have to, interlock your thumbs and let only your fingertips touch the ground. This is a compression pose to massage your pancreas. Remember to keep your breathing relaxed and deep even though your throat is choked. Hold for fifteen seconds, reverse out and repeat the pose on your left side.

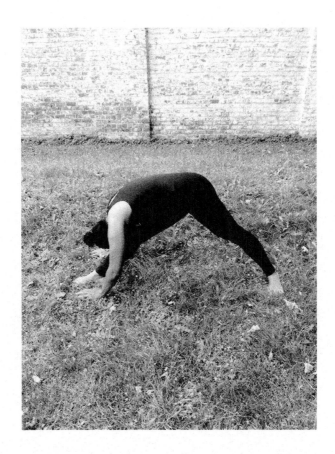

Namaste, your fifteen minutes of Yoga routine for today has now ended. You already finished the exercises for day eight.

For breakfast make a basic fruit smoothie with honey. Bananas are a great way to start the day because they are packed with energizing simple sugars that are easy for your body to digest. They're also packed with potassium which are alkaline forming.

The peaches, mango and strawberries are packed with vitamins and simple sugars that are easy for your body to digest. The simple sugars in honey will give it a sweet kick. Do not skip breakfast. Having woken up in the morning, your body has variable blood sugar, because the last meal you ate was close to twelve hours ago. Having breakfast ensures that your blood-sugar levels are regulated throughout the day.

For lunch you can eat roasted corn and tomato soup with tomato. Tomatoes have a delightful tartness about them and the added spices such as pepper, salt and basil bring it round. You can add just about any of the spices in your spice rack without having to worry about fattening effects. This soup is also a nutritional powerhouse, filled several fat and water-soluble vitamins such as A, E, C and K. It is mainly water. It helps to keep you hydrated through the day.

Tomatoes are rich in antioxidants such as lycopene and carotenoid, two powerhouses in the fight against cancer. Corn contains simple carbohydrates that are easy for the body to digest and give you an energy boost to carry you the day.

At the end of the day have dinner and eat quinoa and garden salad. Containing all the essential amino acids for the human body, quinoa is a complete protein and a good food for new vegetarians who are worried about where to get a reliable source of protein. Seasoning it with black pepper, turmeric and paprika brings the flavor round. Garden Salads are good sources for fiber and you can never go wrong with green, leafy vegetables.

Day eight has been all about your lower abdomen. Before you fall asleep at night lay down on your back, release all the tension in your body, look straight up to the ceiling and think of all the hard work you've done and all the energy you've put into this program. You've done well. This is your time to rest, let your body recover and prepare for day nine.

There you already have your eighth day of healthy living. At the end of the ten days, you can start the program again to make Yoga a part of your daily routine or you can inscribe at www.yogalatinos.com for online classes.

You almost made it!

The 10 DAYS program: Day nine

In a world of instant deliverables, our expectations from a diet are no less different. However, in matters of health, safety is as important as speed. This is why our Yoga exercises and diet to lose 10 pounds in 10 days incorporates generic science behind weight loss.

We are already in day nine of the diet and with one more day to go; your body would have already started to shape up. More importantly, it's beginning to get accustomed to the new lifestyle. So, it's very important to allow the body to transition into accepting this change. A key piece of advice at this stage would be to continue adapting Yoga and healthy meals as a part of your day, permanently.

With that thought, it is recommended that you mix up your exercise a little to create an element of unpredictability. This does not allow the body to get used to a rhythm, thereby increasing the chances of weight loss. Whilst Yoga can be practiced any time of the day, it is most effective between six and eight am when our body metabolism is at a high. One of the keys to effective weight loss has and always be high metabolism. There are three sets of Yoga to be practiced within a fifteen minute span on day nine.

Start the day with a simple breathing technique that involves forceful and rapid inhaling and exhaling. It's called "Kapalbhati".

Exercise 1 – Kapalbhati

This Yoga enables the increase of oxygen in the blood flow. Unlike normal breathing where inhalation is more active, in this Yoga the roles are reversed. Be sure to sit in a steady posture as the breathing momentum creates a vibration in your body that can imbalance you. Further, it's a must that this Yoga is performed on completely empty stomachs. Here follows a step by step guide to Kapalbhati.

Sit upright on a straight spine. After put the hands on your knees. Now breathe in full lungs being completely relaxed. Breathe out in rapid force.When you do this your stomach goes in and towards the thorax to push out stale air from the lungs. Beginners are advised to start with eleven rounds per minute and then increase it to one round per second.

This is a highly effective exercise. But if you suffer from any medical condition please perform the exercise after consent from a medical practitioner.

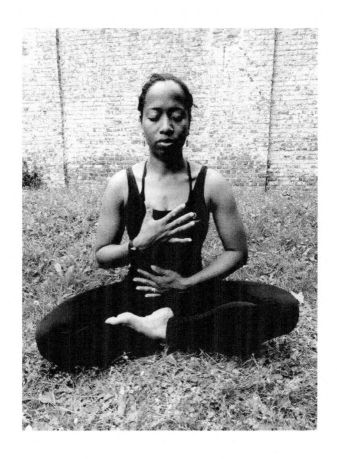

Exercise 2 – The Spine twist

The Spine twist which aids in increasing digestive powers that lead to weight loss. Lie flat on your back. Bring both the knees on your chest. Slowly bring your right leg down and keep it straight. Take your right hand and hold your left knee towards the chest. Bend your left knee across the body while keeping your left hand on the floor. Turn your head towards the left. Hold for about 40 seconds. Repeat on the other side. Do this for about ten minutes. Then take a break for two minutes lying flat on your back

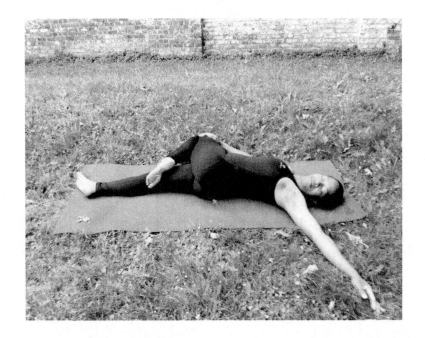

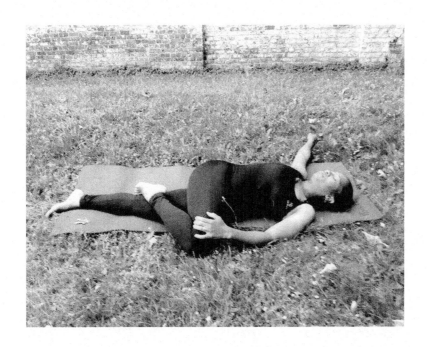

Exercise 3 - The cobra pose

You already know the cobra pose increases metabolism, helps cure stomach disorders and back pain.

Lie on your stomach, making sure your knee joints touch the other. Place your palms near the chest firmly on the ground. Now breathe in and lift only your upper body till your elbows are straight. Bring your head backwards. Hold the position and breath as long as you can. Then slowly start exhaling coming back to the ground, lie flat Beginners can do this 4-5 times

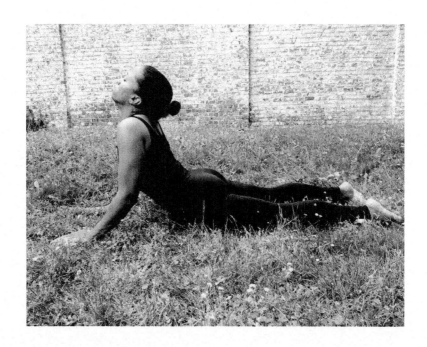

Namaste, your fifteen minutes of Yoga routine for today has now ended. You already finished the exercises for day nine.

Once your three exercises are over, begin the next phase which is your day nine diet, a combination of high proteins, lots of water and inclusion of natural diuretics. Given the exercise regime, your morning meal intake would be the heaviest and subsequently lighten through the day.

One large bowl of unflavored yogurt for breakfast. Two slices of brown bread with some cucumber. A glass of freshly squeezed lime or orange juice for the Vitamin C punch.

Steamed asparagus and spinach with some noodles on the side for lunch. After you can have a cup of green tea and one apple, but only after a 40 minute gap.

For dinner make a bowl of tomato soup flavored with seasonings, using only fresh herbs like celery or parsley as they are natural diuretics. You can also eat cucumber next to it.

For the odd hunger pangs any time of the day eat cucumber and celery only.

If you wish to further reduce your weight, you can repeat our 10 days program. For more tailored results inscribe for Yoga classes at www.yogalatinos.com.

You can do it!
Only one more day to finish the program!

The 10 DAYS program: Day ten

Today is the last day from your 10 days program!
CONGRATULATIONS!
Of course this don't mean that you have to stop here. Let
this 10 days be the start of your new Yoga life.

Go on doing more research, reading, exercises or follow
Yoga classes. Check out www.yogalatinos.com for good
classes, made for you personal. You can follow live classes,
online classes or video classes.

Let us start with the Yoga exercises from our last day of the
10 days program. I'm sure you will go through this day with
a lot of confidence.

Standing Deep-Breathing:
Stand with toes and heels touching. Bring your hands
together and lock your fingers under your chin. Breathe in
deep through your nose and suck your stomach in so that
your ribs are visible. As you breathe in, lift your elbows up
and away from your body as high as they can go, keeping
your knuckles glued to your chin for a count of ten.

Release the breath through your mouth and push your chin up and back with your knuckles until you can see the back of the room that you are in. Let your elbows move forward to touch pointing away from your body. Repeat ten times. This is a great Yoga pose to start the day with as it opens up the lungs, removes stale air and helps to keep the blood oxygenated throughout the day.

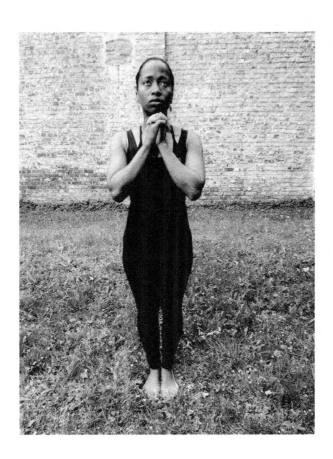

Wind-Removing Pose:

Lay down on your back and lift your right knee. Grip it an inch underneath your knee joint with your fingers interlaced and pull it towards your right shoulder, avoiding the rib cage. Keep the toes on your left leg flexed and pointing towards the ceiling and your left calf muscle touching the ground.

Breath into the pose and you will feel a pinching sensation in your right hip joint. Tuck your chin to your chest and aim your eyes down the center of your body. Pull your knee as close to your shoulder as possible, flexing the muscles in your arms.

Try to keep your entire spine on the ground with each vertebrae from your neck to your coccyx (tail bone) glued to the floor. It will be difficult at first but doing this helps to improve your posture and give you a straight back. This compression pose is great for massaging your descending colon and aids in digestion. Hold in this position for twenty seconds then release and repeat the same posture on your left side. Doing it on your left side massages your ascending colon.

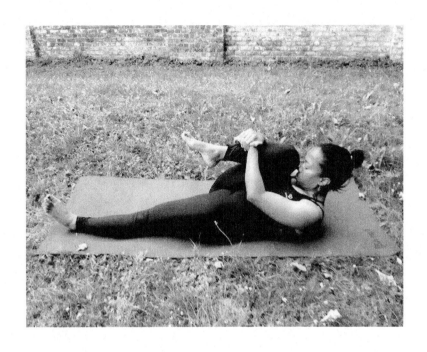

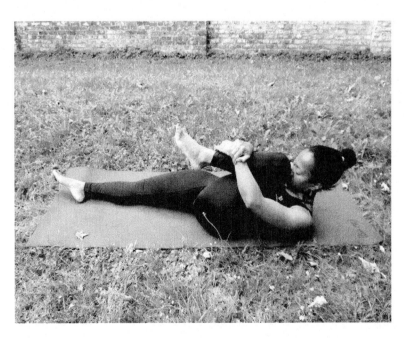

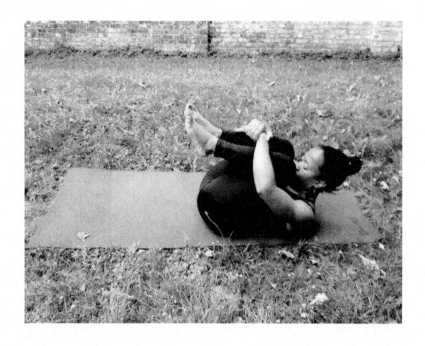

Namaste, your fifteen minutes of Yoga routine for today has now ended. You already finished the exercises for day ten and have now completed all the exercises from the 10 days program.

For breakfast, try a banana, avocado and mango smoothie with peanut butter and coconut oil. Bananas are a great way to start the day because they are packed with energizing simple sugars that are easy for your body to digest. Up to 75% of an avocado's carbs are fiber, making it a low carb friendly plant food.

Peanut butter is an excellent source of protein for vegetarian diets and the coconut oil is great for fat burning as well as boosting your immune system. Do not skip breakfast. Having woken up in the morning, your body has variable blood sugar, the glucose level is higher. This is because the last meal you ate was close to twelve hours ago. Ensuring that you have breakfast ensures that your blood-sugar levels are regulated throughout the day, making it easier to control the urges to overeat.

Tomato soup is perfect for lunch. Tomato soup tastes amazing. Tomatoes have a delightful tartness about them and the added spices such as pepper, salt and basil bring it round. You can add just about any of the spices in your spice rack to your choosing without having to worry about fattening effects.

This soup is also a nutritional powerhouse, filled several fat and water-soluble vitamins such as A, E, C and K. this is one of the most commonly made dishes in India so it's no surprise that they have one of the longest life expectations. It's rich in fiber which is proven to aid in weight loss and as it is mainly water so it helps to keep you hydrated through the day. Tomatoes are also rich in antioxidants such as lycopene and carotenoid, two powerhouses in the fight against cancer.

Enjoy a medium spicy rice noodle salad. While most yogis would suggest to keep to eating a raw diet, eating a cooked meal in has its benefits. Cooked meals don't digest as fast, so you will have a slow release of energy into your bloodstream. Slow digesting foods help you sleep better at night and will keep you from waking up hungry, craving a midnight snack. Try to have your dinner 3-4 hours before bedtime in order to avoid indigestion.

And that's your ten days workout! I'm sure that you loved the program so don't stop there. You can repeat the ten days program and turn healthy living into a part of your everyday lifestyle. For more information and simple everyday Yoga poses, check out the website www.yogalatinos.com or inscribe for Yoga classes.

You are amazing! You made it through the 10 DAYS!
Keep smiling, stay healthy and be blessed!

Chapter 9: What after the 10 DAYS program?

So it has been ten days and maybe you are wondering, what after the 10 days program? Don't worry. This series was about a 10 days plan, but now that you have done this for 10 days, you probably want to continue with some principles, to see what long term health benefits you can have and to continue to keep the healthy and balanced mind and body that you have worked to get in the last ten days.

 By now you understand that Yoga is not just about exercise but a lifestyle choice that has an impact on how you look, how you feel and how you see the world around you. Here are ten tips for how you can continue to experience the benefits you found in the last ten days and keep the positive energy going.

<u>Join a Yoga class:</u>

You now know the basics of Yoga, but with ten days of practice, you are still a beginner. At the early stages, Yoga is often about stretching and if you join a local class and inscribe at www.yogalatinos.com,you will relax and stretch your body, intensively, for 50 minutes to an hour.

Following such a routine about two or three times a week will help you maintain the progress you made in the last ten days. As you move on to advanced levels of Yoga, you will understand that

Yoga routines can offer not only stretching, but also balance, centering of your energy and even strength training, all with none or minimal risk of injury.

Continue to be vegetarian, if possible:

You spent the last ten days either having no meat or very little of it. For some people, this can be very difficult. At this stage, go back to eating little amounts of meat if you want, but you have to reduce the quantity you would normally have and try to continue having salads and lentils too.

You don't have to become a full-fledged vegetarian, but having meat, especially red meat, only as a special treat will be good for your body. And over time, if your body feels right about it, have less and less meat, until it becomes a very rare treat and at that time you will be ready to stop eating meat.

Eat healthy:

You have surely noticed how much better your body has felt in the last few days. This is not only because of what you did from the outside, through exercise, but also because of the change in diet. Once the first ten days are over, you can indulge in a little ice cream or your favorite chips once in a while, but continue to eat mostly fiber-rich, unprocessed food such as leafy vegetables and lentils.

The fiber will help flush out toxins from your body and keeping it functioning healthy. Also continue to avoid foods that are highly processed or rich in salt or sugar. Keep watching your portion size and eat slowly and stop eating before you feel full. It takes your brain some time to realize when the stomach is full and when we eat quickly, we often overeat.

Hydrate:

Continue to start your day with a glass of plain water. If you don't mind the taste, have slightly lukewarm water. Make sure you drink plenty of water throughout the day and that most of the liquids you drink are water. Avoid processed drinks. Some fresh juice is fine, but remember that fruits have lots of natural sugars. It is always better to eat a fruit (with all its fiber content) than to drink lots of juice.

Get enough sleep:

Sleep deprivation can make us unhealthy, leading to physical as well as psychological problems. When we sleep our body works hard, processing the information of the day, repairing damage, fighting illnesses and cleaning out the toxins we gather as we move through life. When you get enough sleep, your body wakes up refreshed and energized. It even shows in your skin!

Maintain a healthy routine:

Some people prefer to stay up late at night while others are happy to wake up early. No matter what your body type is, wake up with enough time for yourself before you have to go to work. Start the day relaxed, so you can calmly plan what you need to do. If you exercise and eat well in the morning, it might be just enough motivation to continue to make healthy choices throughout your day.

Meditate:

Take a few minutes, either early in the day or even sometime later, to sit down, close your eyes and meditate. Take a step back from your life right here and now. This helps to put problems in perspective and make you feel calm and determined about what you need to do in life.

Take time out for nature:

Walk through a park, go for a weekend hike through a forest or even just take care of some potted plants in your balcony or office. City life makes us feel disconnected with nature and reconnecting can be a very soothing experience.

Indulge in ice-cream sometimes:

It's hard to follow very strict rules and breaking them makes us feel guilty. We are human and we all need to indulge sometimes. If your body really wants some ice-cream, have it. Enjoy it!

Love yourself:

You are not perfect, but you are unique and truly special. You work hard on who you are and deserve to be happy about it. Connect with how you feel, be honest with yourself and learn to see all the ways in which you truly are a good person, making a positive impact in the world around you.

The 10 DAYS program is now officially over, but the changes you made to your lifestyle will give you positive benefits for the rest of your life!

Chapter 10: A helping hand for the author

Thank you for purchasing this book and reading it. I hope you will be happy with the results after following the 10 days program. You are now ready to start your journey throughout the Yoga world.

In order to make it possible to do more research and to write more books, it is important to get your full support. You can help a lot by putting some honest reviews on the website from Amazon Kindle. Please keep in mind that by giving a honest five star rate, you will support the author.

If you like the book "How to lose 10 pounds in 10 days with Yoga?", and you want to read more Yoga related books, please check out the other books written by the same author, Sammy Hermans.

Some other titles you will like, are: "How to control your kids with Yoga?", "The Yoga body book", "Happy Yoga", "Loving pregnancy thanks to Yoga" and more coming.

Every time that you buy a book from the author, you are supporting the author to do more research and write more books that can help you in different ways. Every book can give you more insights to Yoga and can help you for a more healthy and happier life. If you have any suggestions or comments, you can report them any time by filling in the contact form at the website www.yogalatinos.com. Please support.

Thanks a lot for the support!

Chapter 11: Thanks and Credits

Thanks to everybody that supported me with writing this Yoga book. Special thanks goes to my partner Sherley Henry De Hermans. She was model for all the Yoga poses and helped with research for the Yoga poses and techniques.

Sherley Henry De Hermans is a Yoga teacher for the company Yoga Latinos and has several years experience with teaching different Yoga styles. She mainly concentrates on Hatha Yoga, Vinyasa Yoga, Ashantha Yoga and Dance Yoga, but she is also an expert in massage and pressure point techniques.

If you are looking for professional help and a perfect guide during your Yoga journey, you can contact Sherley on www.yogalatinos.com for online Yoga classes.

Together we are a Yoga team and we are willing to help you with all your health problems or just getting you to the next Yoga level.

The attitude of gratitude is the highest Yoga.

References

The information in this book was created thanks to the knowledge gained through the years of studying and practicing the Yoga art.

Some of the information and guidelines are created with the knowledge conserved and gained by reading following books:

- *V. Worthington, A History of Yoga, Arkana, London,1982,*

- *S.Swami, Asana Pranayama Mudra Bandha, Yoga Publications Trust,India 2002,*

- *Surendranath, D., A History of Indian Philosophy, Cambridge University Press, 1955,*

- *G. Feuerstein, The Yoga Tradition, Hohm Press, Arizona, 2001.*

The true method of knowledge is experiment.

Extra bonus

Because I am so happy that you were reading all of my book, I will give you the first chapter from my book "How to control your kids with Yoga?" completely FREE so you can already enjoy it.

Chapter 1: Can this book really help me ?

Raising children the right way is considered to be one of the most challenging tasks in the world. Common phrases such as 'lioness mum' has made way into many children's vocabulary. When your child is out of control, the most reasonable action to take would be over-parenting through keeping curfews, punishments and grounding.

Most parents couple this with no allowances. All of the parents have the same questions about their children. The million dollar question is; can this book really help me (with controlling kid)? The answer is, **YES!**

While many mothers may think that over emphasizing the parental elbow grease may assure their children of great futures, this may not be the right way to go. It hardly is. This may just make our children that much more distant from us. Truth is when your child is out of control, parental involvement through friendly ways may be the solution. The most friendly being Yoga; a practice that is always considered overrated and often under estimated.

According to statistics, 67% of mothers have been able to save their troubled children by signing them up for Yoga. When mothers use Yoga to parent, it easily eliminates the continuum between authoritarian and permissive parenting. Yoga offers a great alternative that we often dismiss. Generally, through it, many mothers learn how to listen and communicate with their troubled kids. It's a mindful and conscious ways to communicate.

You may be wondering, can this book really help me when it comes to your troublesome child? Provided you are open-minded and are willing to accept other practical ways to fine tune your parenting and care for your child then this is the right book for you.

The first step in embarking on this journey is usually self-acceptance. When we accept our kids as they are then we begin accepting help with our parental ways.

Asking yourself can this book really help me, should no longer be a question of worry. The only valid question in your mind as a mother at this point should be where to start with Yoga. It is a practice that has been dated but still never loses its value. Many will raise better children academically, psychologically and socially.

For one thing, Yoga will help any mother cultivate motivation in their child as well as instill some wisdom in their parenting. When your child accesses the most integral part of their body, they also become one with their mind and spirit. Yoga is an ideal solution when it comes to the pursuit of inner harmony. When your child is out of control, they often create this exterior that may not really allow you to get through to them.

However, Yoga will provide a platform that will encourage them to deal with their emotional conflicts and challenges. Slowly, they will learn how to react to situations, understand self- discovery and be more inquisitive about the things that make them happy. It's a rare opportunity for any troublesome child to do participate in something without being told that they are wrong.

The other benefits are tremendous; as a parent, you obviously want to be present throughout your child's challenges and vulnerabilities. For a child who is out of control even more, Yoga will enable them to face everyday difficulties with ease. They don't have to end up at the curb or at a detention center. Even if they do change their lifestyle in this way, it will ensure that they do not return to their behavioral pattern. The idea behind it is to provide children and growing with viable options that they can use as tools to change their lives.

Mums have the toughest job in the world. Yoga may make it a little easier. It transcends everything into a more constructive and happier place. Needless to say, your child will acquire feelings of competency, gain inner strength, and have extra determination and a higher sense of optimism. On the other hand, if your child somehow ended up in a correctional center, you need not to despair. 65% of teenagers in such places are participating in a daily Yoga program. This serves as a peaceful coping mechanism for them.

From a physical standpoint, Yoga enhances flexibility and refines coordination. It develops muscular structure and promotes good physical shape. Apart from getting the emotional support that your child needs to stay in control, Yoga is also beneficial to their physical health.

Asking yourself; "can this book really help me?" should be a question that's dead and gone. Mindful meditation can benefit a troubled child by not only empowering them but also encouraging them to look before they leap. This is a great strategy to self-control.

When we think of Yoga, the image of a child that's out of control and probably needs help does not really spring to mind. That's why only you can understand the difficulties that you are facing with your child and you are the only one that can remedy it.

In a typical experiment, children of different ages and from different backgrounds were asked to solve a simple Lego puzzle. Usually, difficult puzzles are known to separate the 'smart and confident' kids from the rest in the bunch. What the 'smart and confident' children did not know is that the rest of the group was more motivated to tackle the puzzle. So is Yoga; it motivates and turns things around when you least expect it. The experiment also confirmed what most mums tend to forget: "your child will be happier and more successful when you do things that satisfy their own needs; even if they are capable of doing it on their own".

The sole purpose of this book is to indulge your out of control child and help them to develop a sense of self that is autonomous, confident and generally in accord with reality. This book will most definitely let you have control over your out of control child. With the best Yoga practices, they will certainly be on the straight and narrow. This book will not only account for behavioral changes through Yoga but will also elevate your parenting to a solid ten.

Yes, you and your kids can do this!

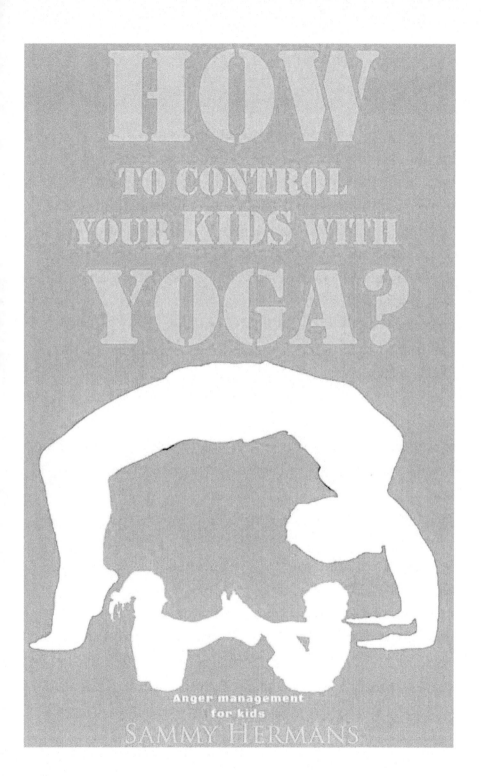

Book tags

yoga, yoga for beginners, yoga diet, stress relief, meditation, beginners, inner peace, mindfulness, Yoga, anxiety, mood management, Restore the balance, weight loss guide, stress, books, mindfulness meditation, yoga guide, meditation for beginners, meditation books, yoga books, zen meditation, how to meditate, ashtanga yoga, hatha yoga, vinyasa yoga, self-help, increase productivity, daily meditations, yoga for weight loss, relieve stress, yoga anatomy, spiritual growth, yoga stress relief, yoga, yoga for beginners, yoga for meditation, helpful books, books for life, health books, diet, asana, ashtanga, bhakti, Buddha, drishti, guru, karma, karuna, kula, prana, agami karma, sun salutation, standing poses, balancing poses, sitting poses, halasana, salamba sarvangasana, tadasana, utkatasana, ustrasana, savasana, boat pose, bow pose, bridge pose, basic poses, utkatasana, modified downward facing dog, warrior pose, half moon pose, sun, motivation, groving, veight loss every day, training program, diet books, healthy living, outdoor, yoga at home, meditation for stress relief, tired, yoga for women, advanced Yoga, energy, active, yoga for beginners, healthy food, detox, diet plan, organic food, overweight, feel better, motivate yourself, diet program that helps, yoga books for beginners, yoga, weight loss book, losing weight thanks to yoga, meditation outside, happy, family, teaching, coaching, relax, relaxation, kids yoga, yoga for women above 50, yoga for advanced, yogi, better life, younger, health benefits, impove, more, no more damage, food choices, veggie, vegetarian, diet for weight loss, yoga world, yoga classes, yoga for pregnant women, yoga for baby's, yoga all day, thanks, mudras, mudras for beginners, chakras, chakras for advanced, meditation for beginners, mind, body, soul, spirit, light, heart, feelings, good, great, yoga love, healthy mind, mind-control, yoga breathing, breath controlling, becoming young again, youth, yoga spirit, yoga journey, music, yoga music, yoga mood, yoga meditations, yoga for yogi, food that is good, happy food, yoga happy food, important, self-awareness, self-doubts, relationship, practicing yoga, panic attacks, discipline, strenght, increase health, deeper wisdom, burn fat fast, burn belly fat, yoga diet book, yoga health program, yoga results, yoga beginner, improve memory, memory training, brain power, blood pressure, cardio, alertness, yoga forever, yoga symbols, cure, yoga basic poses, yoga in the morning, yoga breakfast, yoga cadio, yoga for weight loss book, yoga diet program, yoga, diet food, energy food, growing up with yoga, yoga for weight problems, feel good yoga, yoga mental power, yoga inner peace, yoga body, yoga cures, yoga systems for weight loss, lose weight fast, yoga energy, yoga breath control, yoga course, yoga peace, yoga program for health problems,yoga, yogi

Printed in Great Britain
by Amazon

10336299R00088